STORIES OF CHANGING LIVES 3

CONTENTS & ARTWORKS

FOREWORD

*'And she, remembering other things, to me trifles
but torturing to her, showed me how life withers when
there are things that we cannot share.'*

The Waves, Virginia Woolf

It is an honour to have been asked by the Management Committee of
the Patients' Council to provide this foreword in memory of my Dad,
Ronnie Jack, who died in December 2016. Ronnie had volunteered
within the Royal Edinburgh Hospital for 20 years. He was elected
to the Management Committee of the Patients Council in 2010 and
served as its Convener in 2012, and its Vice Chair in 2015.

I have neither lived experience of mental illness, nor am I a mental
health care professional, so it is with a degree of trepidation that I add
my voice to the courageous contributors who follow. I hope, however,
to tell a bit of 'our story': the story of my Dad, for whom there were
periods when each day was an internal battle, and of those of us who
walked alongside him during those times.

First, I want to pay tribute to the contribution that Ronnie made to
this ever-evolving Changing Lives Project by taking the helm of the
good ship *Stories of Changing Lives II* in 2014 and steering it safely to
its publication the following year. As well as editing all the content, he
co-ordinated others to deliver the many other aspects of publication,
including the illustrations and design. Indeed, my Mum would perhaps
argue, he took the role a bit too far, when he agreed that the full print
run could be delivered to their house. But, then, he didn't do things
half-heartedly; he believed passionately in the value of the Changing

Lives concept, and the second volume is a lasting testament to this. But relying on one volunteer, who just happened to have such a unique blend of skills, drive and time, to keep Changing Lives going was clearly unsustainable, and Ronnie was delighted when the Council secured dedicated funding for Katherine. He felt this was an important step in recognising the value of this project, and was keen to see what form its third metamorphosis would take under her care.

Second, I wish to acknowledge that my Dad's work on *Changing Lives II* was all done during a time when our family's life had been impacted once more by the recurring thoughts that had, unfortunately, started to dominate his outlook again. My Mum, sister and I were witness to a man, who we loved dearly - and who had, without doubt, achieved and contributed so much in both his personal and professional life – start to battle with questions of his own worthiness. We sat with him as he ruminated on thoughts which, when well, would have caused him no more than a fleeting tinge of anxiety. We would even converse with these thoughts, because – just every now and then – we could persuade them to quieten sufficiently to allow my Dad's true voice to ring out again and his peace of mind to return. And, through it all, we watched him continue to give of his own time to make a positive difference to the lives of others, including providing invaluable mentoring support to fellow members of the Patients' Council.

When I look back on our experience, I often return to the words of a wise woman who told me that while you cannot take away another person's suffering, you can make it more bearable. My Dad inherently knew that there is a common basic need in us all to feel that we are heard and understood - and that such support can make all the difference during hard times. Moreover, while we may never be able to fully understand how it feels to walk in someone else's shoes, he believed that the very act of trying would bring us closer. But, if no one has the courage to tell their story, then there is nothing to hear and our opportunity to increase our connection with others reduces. So, it is for this reason that – like my Dad did before me - I consider the Changing Lives volumes to be so vital.

Ronnie ended his introduction to *Changing Lives II* hoping that the quality of its content would encourage support for *Changing Lives III*. He would be delighted not only that it did, but that this third volume continues the series in such a vibrant, inclusive and creative way. The credit for this goes to Katherine for taking over the helm so successfully, and to all those who have contributed. In the pages that

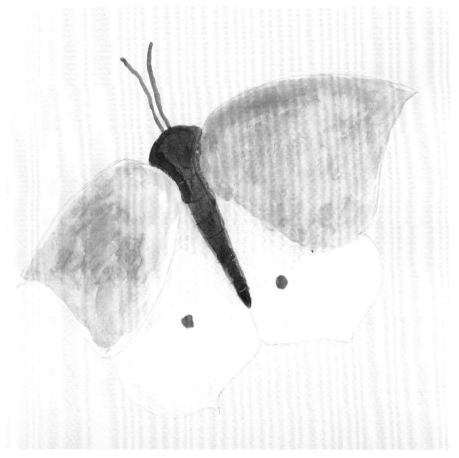

Anna Redpath, *From chrysalis to flight*

follow, people have shared their experiences of mental health with the same courage as in previous volumes, while again the project continues to evolve from one publication to the next.

Photographs now join the poetry and narratives, other animals jostle alongside the butterflies and all appear within a larger format. They invite an emotional response from us, offering a chance to better understand one another and providing the perfect springboard for *Changing Lives IV*. As such, this volume is a precious gift indeed.

Isla Jack

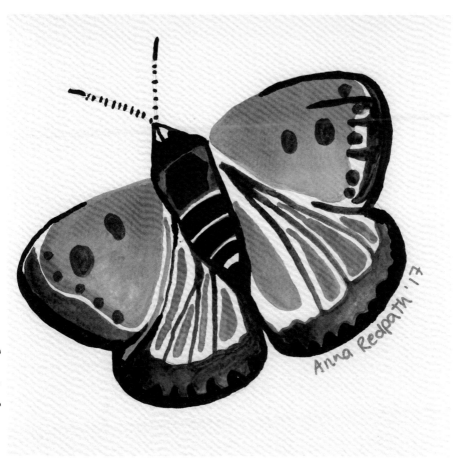

Anna Redpath, *Orangina*

INTRODUCTION

Welcome to the third volume of Stories of Changing Lives!

The series collects together the stories and artwork of people who have spent time in the Royal Edinburgh Hospital. The contributors describe their journeys from hospital to community – journeys which are not always in straight lines, and which are often still in progress. They generously take us with them so that we can learn from their experiences: the book aims to be a source of support and solidarity for those who are on similar journeys, and a resource for professionals, family, friends, and members of the public who want to understand mental ill health better.

The Patients Council is a collective advocacy organisation based at the Royal Edinburgh. It is run by patients and former patients, with the aim of strengthening patients' voices and improving the hospital and its services. This book is part of that mission: by providing a platform for these stories, the hospital will be able to learn about what works and what doesn't from the viewpoint of those who use its services. It is also a tool for fighting the stigma around mental health and psychiatric hospital admission more widely, through a deeper understanding and a sense of connection with these experiences.

This is possible because of the huge creativity and talent of the contributors to this book. Art has the ability to express something that case studies and medical notes can't: you will put this book down with a greater understanding of what it feels like to be a patient. You will find experiences in this book that you won't hear about anywhere else, from the people who are the experts on the journey.

The book focuses on the experiences of people who have had longer stays in hospital – on the rehabilitation or forensic wards, through longer stays in acute wards, or through several admissions. They have a huge amount of knowledge about what does and doesn't work, and how things have changed, as well as their own experience of the journey.

This book is the third in a series, and owes a debt to those who produced and contributed to the previous volumes. The series has evolved over the years – from the interviews of book one, to the addition of poetry in book two, to the multimedia volume that you hold in your hands right now. The first two books were produced by volunteers, who worked amazingly hard to make the project happen. This new stage was made possible by funding from NHS Lothian's Mental Health Strategy, A Sense of Belonging, which enabled the Patients Council to employ me three days a week for eight months, as well as bringing in a photographer, a film-maker, and a social history element – making the project bigger and more diverse than would have otherwise been possible.

Having a variety of ways to be part of the project meant that contributors could choose how they want to tell their story, supporting more people to be involved:

For those who express themselves best through writing, contributors could submit written pieces – whether poetry or prose – with the offer of support in the process. I ran creative writing and storytelling workshops to offer some inspiration and to let people know about the project. These sessions were hugely enjoyable, and it was a joy to work with such talented and imaginative people, whether or not they decided to contribute work to the book in the end.

For those who feel most comfortable speaking their stories (and I had the privilege of hearing from some amazing storytellers!), they could do an informal interview with me, and/or be part of the film that accompanies this book, produced by Peter E. Ross of Chiaroscuro. The interviews were transcribed, and I edited them for length and flow – with the contributors getting final say. Some of the interviews include my questions to give a sense of the conversation, while some of them worked better as uninterrupted stories.

For those who express themselves visually, there was the option to work on photography with Margaret Drysdale, or take part in art workshops with Anne Elliot at Artlink. The previous books included a butterfly motif; for this edition, we decided to broaden out with a prompt that takes in the whole animal kingdom: the artists were asked to create work based on an animal that represents an emotion present in their mental health journey; the results are evocative and eclectic. We have a few butterflies fluttering through the book as well, providing a visual link to the previous books and paying tribute to the evolution of Stories of Changing Lives. This prompt was just a suggestion, so there is also some artwork which provides a different angle.

As with previous volumes, we asked staff to contribute their experiences of working in the hospital. An occupational therapist, two third sector workers, a peer worker, and a clinical nurse specialist all generously agreed to be part of the book; their voices join with patients and ex-patients to give an extra dimension to the journey from hospital to community.

The final facet of the project is the work done by CAPS Independent Advocacy staff and volunteers. They carried out a series of interviews which captured stories of people making change happen at the Royal Edinburgh Hospital, from seemingly small improvements to services, to the recent repro-visioning of the hospital. The piece People Make Change presents excerpts of the transcripts and the full collection of stories will become part of the organisations 'Oor Mad History' archive. The groundwork for this strand was laid by Lili Fullerton, and the final work was created by Pam van de Brug. People Make Change joins some of the other pieces in calling for people with lived experience of mental ill health to be listened to, believed, and treated as the experts that they are. This section is a testament to the strength and power of mental health activists, and we hope it will be inspiring and empowering for future change.

This book is being produced at a time of huge change, as phase one of the new hospital opens up, and phase two gears up to renovate Mackinnon House. This change is reflected throughout the book: excitement and hope at the provision of single en suite rooms with views onto green spaces – which will have a huge impact on the experience of being in hospital – as well as reflections on the process.

This sense of space is a strong theme in many pieces. Having a space to just be, has a profound impact on many of the contributors, whether that's a quiet spot in the hospital grounds, the importance of having a private room, or the joy of making a home.

An image that really struck me, in 'Keys', was the hope of having family over to your own house for dinner as a really important moment in the journey. Family is another theme which comes up a lot in the book – and contributors' experience of this is as complicated and varied as families themselves. Families provide essential support and love, and several contributors pay moving tribute to the importance of their family. The other side of this coin is that when things are not so good – when bereavements or estrangements break connections – it can be extremely painful, and can have an effect on mental health.

This sense of connection is a really key part of the way people stay well. Whether connections with families, friends, faith communities, or peer support – there is a strong message throughout the book that kindness, solidarity, understanding, and listening are incredibly important.

Volunteering contributes to these connections: it links people into communities and creates opportunities to do work that brings satisfaction and joy. Several contributors talk about the hugely positive effect that volunteering has had on their lives, and many highlight the importance of purpose and meaningful activities – including creative ones – as essential to their journey and their ongoing wellbeing. They emphasise that clinical intervention such as medication, while important, is only a part of what people need to be well.

Which brings us full circle to art: as advocacy, as solidarity, as fulfilment, simply as creativity. This book is a piece of art and a historical artefact as well as a resource; it celebrates the talent, strength, and diversity of people who are or have been patients at the Royal Edinburgh.

We hope it will give you insight, understanding, solidarity, and hope.

Katherine McMahon
Editor and Stories of Changing Lives Development Worker, 2017

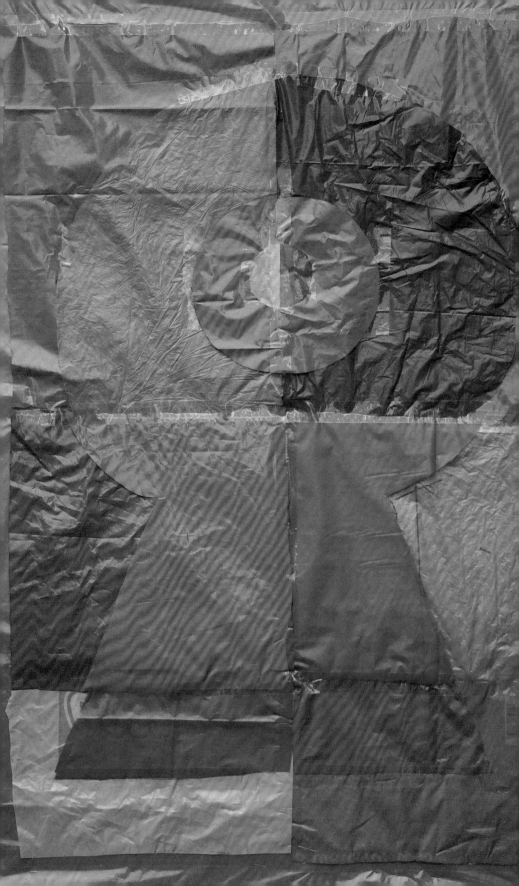

Content warnings:

This book discusses experiences of mental ill health, and of psychiatric hospital admission. Because some people might find it difficult to read about certain topics, we have included a list of the pieces in which common triggers come up. We would encourage you to take care of your emotional wellbeing while reading this book: take a break when you need to, discuss anything you find difficult if you can, and if it does bring up any issues for you, please seek support. If you need to talk to someone, you can always call the Samaritans free on 116 123.

◦ Discussion of mental health issues throughout
◦ Suicide: 'Paranoia – a perspective lost', 'My experience of madness', 'Don't use drugs', 'Hell-in-a-cell', 'Drawing strength from one another', 'Never give up'
◦ Psychosis / delusions / hearing voices: 'My experience of madness', 'Don't use drugs', 'Horrible moments to home comforts', 'Home', 'Hell-in-a-cell'
◦ Drug use: 'Don't use drugs', 'Hell-in-a-cell', 'Never give up'
◦ Violence: 'Don't use drugs', 'Hell-in-a-cell'
◦ Bereavement: 'Horrible moments to home comforts', 'Home', 'Hell-in-a-cell', 'Never give up'
◦ Rape: 'Hell-in-a-cell'
◦ Self harm: 'Hell-in-a-cell', 'Drawing strength from one another'
◦ Racism: 'Hell-in-a-cell'
◦ Abuse: 'Hell-in-a-cell'
◦ Cults: 'Hell-in-a-cell'

JOHN

Paranoia - a perspective lost

I was born in Edinburgh. I had a pretty happy upbringing; I had a loving family. My mother was from a pretty poor background, but the one thing about the family was – no matter how poor they were, they still showed respect of things around them.

At primary school I was one of the best players on the football pitch. I was also the school sprinter – I was the one that could outrun anybody. It was me and a girl, blue-eyed, blonde hair. The two of us were like champions together.

I went to secondary school, and that's where some problems started, because there was an element within the school that had decided that they would bully some of the other pupils. As the years went on I decided that there was a little bit more respect shown for me. At the end of the day, things actually worked out not too badly, although I did have a great fear of flunking exams.

I went on to go into college and I studied for a degree in engineering. It was only at college that I began to realise there are many different techniques for studying for exams.

I realised that sometimes it's not the detail that's important; sometimes it's the way you approach something that's important.

I came top of the class on several occasions. My final-year project was a satellite dish position control system, and I took off like a rocket – I'll tell you, I loved it. From there, I applied for three jobs and I got two job offers; I became a combat systems development engineer in Barrow. That was pretty good fun.

One of the guys in the office introduced me to the president of the amateur dramatics society, who was also in charge of the set building. Colin introduced a whole new aspect to my life that I'd never really considered.

We used to go up to this big barn and do the set building. There was a welder, there was a butcher, there was a painter, there was myself – an engineer – and there was Colin, who was a pharmacist.

We had a lot of camaraderie. It was good fun.

I did that with them for a year or two. When I saw what they were doing onstage, I thought, "Maybe I could have a shot at this." Colin got more and more encouraging that I should go for one of the roles, so I went for the part of Georgie Locke from London. It was a sell-out show. We had rehearsed a great deal, and it was just like going into an exam where you knew what the questions were, but could you keep your brain in gear to get those answers written?

The show went on, and it got a standing ovation. At the end of the day, I thought it was a job well done. I didn't get big-headed about it, but I enjoyed it.

That night my sisters, and brother-in-law, and my mum and dad, and all the cast were partying in the auditorium.

Things started to go wrong because I was kept up all night partying - not drinking all that much, but just partying. I was exhausted.

Then I had to show my brother-in-law and sister around Barrow, because they were interested in the shipyard area. When they left, I parked my car at the back of the flat and went into the flat just for a rest and a cup of tea. When I came back out of the flat, my car had been broken into. I thought, "Okay, I've got insurance, I can replace it."

A few days later, there were some incidents below my flat and I couldn't understand what was going on. It involved the car, and I phoned the police and I said to them, "There are some really strange things going on. I think you should come round and have a look."

I had noted down everything as much as I possibly could to give the police a statement, and the police turned round to me and said, "Was it a police car you saw?" I said, "What? A police car? You've got to be kidding. If it was a police car, why in the bloody hell would I have phoned the police?"

That was where the start of the paranoia began, and that just went from one thing to another.

I started to see people looking at me all the time, and I just got wound up and wound up, and I was sent on four or five weeks' sick leave. When I came back I settled down into work, but I couldn't concentrate properly.

Since I've signed the 'Official Secrets Act', I can't say much more about it after that, but I came back to Edinburgh in 1994, having just attempted suicide, driving a car at 96mph into a stone wall. I've got scars on my head to prove it.

I was only in hospital two days. I got my wounds stitched up as soon as I got into hospital, and one woman said to me, "You're a very brave man." I said to myself, "You don't know how brave I am," because I'm not telling anybody that I've just attempted suicide because I was sick and tired of being put on locked wards. They were just a sheer bloody hell.

I had been in two hospitals in Lancaster. If you think about the jail in 'Porridge', you might get some idea of the austerity of the buildings. It put fear into anybody, so the fact is I hated the bloody places.

I didn't tell anybody, but, when I came back from hospital after my mum and dad picked me up, my dad had turned round to me and said, "John, have you just attempted suicide?" I said, "Aye." He said, "I knew that was the case. I knew you were too good a driver to do that sort of thing."

You know something? I didn't

admit to anybody, apart from my parents. I didn't even tell my sisters or friends. I was charged with careless driving; I got a £48 fine, 5 points on my licence, and I passed my motorcycle test first time that same year.

I'm a man, as an engineer, who loves to work machinery of any sort, and I have some connection between my brain and my body about how to do anything with that. I could drive anything; I really could.

I came back to Edinburgh, got involved in a bit of rehabilitation. I did that at a unit in Edinburgh who had a clerk. She needed some help to put together a computer programme to do the statistics for her side of the ward management. She asked me if I could help out. I put it together, and got it working, to her delight.

At the end of the day they said, "Thanks, we think you're becoming too dependent on the unit, so bugger off," more or less. I wasn't dependent on the unit at all. They were dependent on me to do the job.

Anyway, I liked a lot of the people there – some really good occupational therapists, which is one of the most important parts of recovery. After being at the unit, there was a transition into the community with the same occupational therapist, doing pottery and joinery. It was great fun.

I come from an artistic family. My sister was having an exhibition, and at that exhibition I met this man who was doing metal sculpture at Telford College and starting a new course. He had been a professional welder.
We got on really pretty well and he said, "Come along. Have an interview; see what you're interested in."

It was a springboard onto something else - another thing that really occupied me and that I enjoyed.

I got an HNC in public art and I got a merit. The welded metal sculpture was my speciality, and I sold £2,500 worth of objects in one exhibition.

It was money that really the government should have given me.

I had Disability Living Allowance 10 years too late because, when I first applied for it, I didn't want to admit that I'd attempted suicide. My CPN eventually convinced me that that was the approach.
To hell with the bloody benefit people. They make you slaves to the system. I earned just enough money to buy my wife-to-be an engagement ring and to buy a motorbike, and that's all I really wanted.

I had a happy relationship with my wife. She had mental health problems and I had mental health problems. When I first met her, I took her to a classic car show in my classic car, and when we got home from the show we were discussing each other's problems and she said to me, "I've got agoraphobia." I said, "You've got agoraphobia and you've gone all the way to Selkirk with me? How the hell did you manage that?" She said to me, "I had so much trust in you that I knew that if I was ill you'd turn back." I said, "Bloody hell. That shows a lot of trust in somebody that you hardly know," because that was one of our first dates.

We got on really well. I met the family, and met her friends.

We were in each other's company almost 24/7, and I did a lot of support for her.

It was difficult at times because she couldn't always see my point of view, my illness. There was once that she accused me of coming into hospital just because she had physical ailments and this was me getting back at her. That wasn't true at all. It was just because I was so worried about her that it was affecting my mental health.

In 2009 my father died. Shortly afterwards I went into hospital in Livingston. Shortly after that, I had a blowout argument with my wife and told her, "You can have that divorce if you want it," and she took it. I thought, "Fair enough," and in hospital I thought I could deal with it. Everything else was happening to me anyway and it was difficult to concentrate on any one thing.

When I got home, I was starting to miss her. She moved out, but she was within a mile of where I lived, so occasionally I was able to have a coffee with her, but that was about it. Eventually, we even got out of the habit of texting.

Things have changed again. I've just been involved in a house move which was quite stressful, which has brought me into hospital, but I now feel that my feet are firmly planted on the ground. My experience here in the hospital has been really interesting. Other patients on my ward have come to me to write their notes and hand those notes into the doctors, and the nurses, and the advocacy service, and the lawyers. We just cover all the bases so that the notes can't go missing for some reason – everybody that we can think of, including family members. That's where the battle is, and that's where you identify people who don't want you to recover, who milk the system for the money and aren't interested in helping people to recover. I didn't go into engineering to earn millions of pounds; I went into engineering because I loved to build things and understand how they worked.

The other patients have helped me. We have banded together. We are shipmates on board a ship.

We get on so well – we can have such a laugh. A lot of the nurses are joining in and have a great time. There are one or two blank canvases of doctors, but we just ignore them as much as possible.

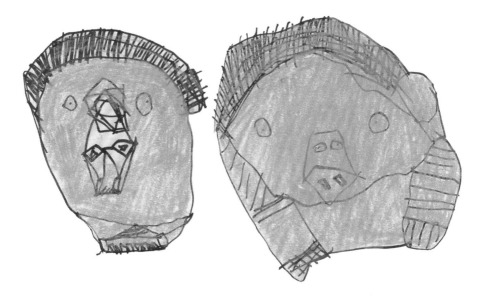

In the meantime, we communicate with the SHOs – they're interested in learning.

A holistic point of view for recovery is about involving all sorts of professions. It's just opening your eyes.

The simple things can be the best solutions; natural things can be the best cures.

Some of the growing spaces in this hospital, and just the beautiful grounds and the way they've nurtured the new hospital – there's going to be a lot of recovery with the right people helping. Not only that, though: I said to the hospital planners,

"Don't make the place too sterile. Otherwise, there'll never be recovery." I said, "Why don't you have hospital radio? Why don't you have stimulation on the ward? Why don't you get the damn government to stop all this bed blocking? Why don't you get more support in people's houses so that they can cope with their disabilities in their own homes?"

The government have got to change from this superior power to being one that cares for its people. Industries can be driven by caring for people, and people will be driven to those industries, and the world will be a much happier and more peaceful place.

SIMON

Sovereign Rings

In a second or two, you may feel a sharp prick,
But please, don't you worry, it's over so quick:

Twinsets and pearls will come at a price;
Tracksuits and sovvies will make you think twice.

HOLLY C. BEHAN

My experience of Madness

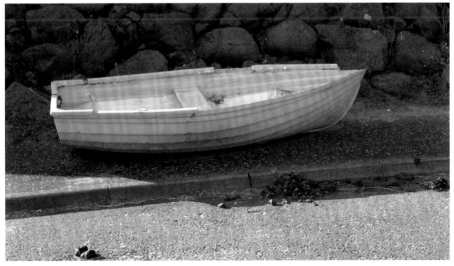

Holly C. Behan, *Boat*

Originally a Photovoice project - an exploration of image and experience - for the Mad People's History Course at Queen Margaret's University

It took me a while to choose this photograph to depict my experience of psychosis, as initially when I took the snap it was because I simply liked the colour of the boat and just perceived it as a pretty picture – ideal to put up in my bathroom. However, as I started to look through my other photos which depicted fairly obvious images of distress (for example, ones of myself looking very depressed indeed), I found myself always returning to the image above. As I reflected on my psychological distress prior to my emergency hospital admission, I realised that this photograph of the stranded boat very much illustrated my experience, and could be used to dispel some of the myths surrounding the perception of 'Madness' and in particular, psychosis. The Stereotype of 'Madness' contains images of mania, chaos, severe agitation and destructive behaviour. Such phrases as "eyes out on stalks" or "dribbling at the mouth" are not uncommon in the Media and the Public.

However, the image I chose above resonates with my experience of 'Madness' of being isolated, lonely, threatened, helpless and absolutely terrified. I had managed to function to an acceptable degree but then 'something went'! In the image, the little green boat is damaged and neglected in appearance. It has run aground and stuck with no oars to steer away from danger or towards safety and, probably most significantly, is missing a boatman! I felt this was happening to me.

I was 'disappearing' and was worried that I would finally have to 'bail out'.

However, there is a sense that this image is acceptable. It is a calm scene and does not necessarily resound of imminent danger. We have an idea that this static situation can be easily remedied with a lick of paint, some repair to the structure, some oars and with a few hands to carry it back to the sea. This, I now believe, is what people perceived in me. They were not listening to understand that without a well and confident captain on-board to restore order, the picture was incomplete and I was doomed to fail. I was receiving counselling and a tweak to my medication was thought to be enough, despite the fact I was convinced my medication was making me feel this way! So instead of reviewing my medication, the dosage was increased to the maximum!

This is how my meltdown felt. With no other options to try, my familiar mind 'turned off' and metaphorically abandoned ship! All that we consider as human qualities such as: emotion; hope; a desire to live and have purpose in life; morality and awareness of the consequences of our action – all seemed to leave consciousness. What replaced it seemed to be pure reason that operated in a vacuum from the aforementioned measures to deal with the pain and terror I felt.

With this massive force crushing me and threatening obliteration, to wait any longer became impossible.

Starting from the premise that I had to die ASAP, my mind made cold calculations to do the "right thing" and hasten my death to end the terror. Thus, the last automatic response left was FLIGHT when I eventually leapt from my window, as the

FIGHT was lost. The captain of that boat had abandoned ship with psychosis leading the way. When I regained consciousness from incomplete suicide, I was completely heartbroken as I had destroyed the life I had cherished so much before my mental ill-health took over!

Why could I not have been helped before tragedy struck?

Although this happened one night, the build up to it was a gradual process. I had asked for help many times and discussed with psychiatric professionals how desperate and scared I felt. However, I was constantly told "you're ok", "don't worry, you're coping better than you think" and "you need to reduce your stress levels".

Each time I tried to express my concern that something was severely wrong and that I felt different from ever before, I was rebuffed as being "wrong in my assessment of the situation". I expressed concern about my medication but each time I failed to convince them that "I knew something was very wrong with my mind", something majorly frightening was happening and that I was "beginning to disappear". I believe people, like myself, saw a similar kind of picture in me as the 'little green boat' and assumed everything was basically ok and salvageable. I did not fit the image of 'mad person'.

On the surface I seemed OK (like I initially felt about the image of the boat) and still functioning, so my account of my experience could not be trusted. I was not believed when I said I could not cope for much longer. Eventually, when I was in utter crisis and sought emergency help, I was persuaded that hospital was not the answer from someone who had a very difficult experience with hospitalisation and believed I wouldn't cope.

A fear of services was the last straw to an already terrified mind on top of not being heard. How could all this have been avoided?

Many academics have acknowledged these anomalies. Peter Beresford (Brunel University, Middlesex UK), has written extensively on the value of 'survivor knowledge' and the importance of the service user being an 'expert by experience.' In the Journal of Mental Health (2002) 11, 6, 581-584, (Article: Thinking about 'mental health': towards a social model), Beresford argues that philosophy has hardly changed since the 19th Century model of mental health, unlike other areas of medicine. He reviews the political and policy context within mental health, and the emergence within this of 'survivor knowledge' that draws on the standpoint of those with first-hand experience of mental distress and of the impact of services upon them.

He also addresses the problem of the lack of investment in good mental health services for the vast majority of service users who do not 'pose a public threat'. This means that more funds are available for Forensic Services which is quite obviously too little, too late for patients and society! This is not only backward financial thinking but also socially bankrupting. A change in attitudes towards mental health and its sufferers has to happen!

I spent many years in a Forensic ward and can testify to the above. I met people in a very similar position to me as well as those who had been released from a main hospital too early 'whilst begging to stay an inpatient' as they knew they were still very ill. Ironically, the service there was excellent with person centred care from a multidisciplinary team who are there for you every step of the way. They are there to catch you if you slip back but also there to help you plan and realise your goals.

The Forensic unit was so much nicer than any other psychiatric service I had visited relatives in before, with single rooms, lots of light and plenty of therapies to occupy the long days.

However, the restrictions required in such a service can be degrading and humiliating. Also, at times, it could be even more difficult to have your word believed as now you were not only 'mad' but also 'bad' and thus to be treated with suspicion. However, over time (which was in abundance), I started to gradually recover some dignity and self-belief with the help of psychological therapy and some excellent staff.

A combination of crisis in Mental Health provision and understanding have life and death consequences, namely: underinvestment leading to a lack of beds and time to help people recover some skills and confidence to manage the symptoms of a difficult illness; trust in the service user's voice; and lastly a rigidity in the system unable to treat patients as individuals with very different needs.

Encouragingly, a credible challenge to the dominant psychiatric ideology now exists in the form of the mental health service user/survivor movement. Since the mid-1980s this movement has been gaining strength and reputation.

More psychiatric professionals are beginning to break from the mould and trying to listen to us. For the main, there is a missing link between the professionals and the patient, and that is the patient's voice of experience.

I have now decided to join this movement in the hope that services and their reputation can be improved for all stakeholders and society at large. We can all learn from each other by coming to the table as equal partners to share our respective expertise. Service users need to be given back control of their situation with the help of others to make meaningful recovery possible.

Invictus (extract)

William Ernest Henley

Out of the night that covers me,
    Black as the pit from pole to pole,
   . . . .
I am the master of my fate,
    I am the captain of my soul.

MAGGIE KEPPIE

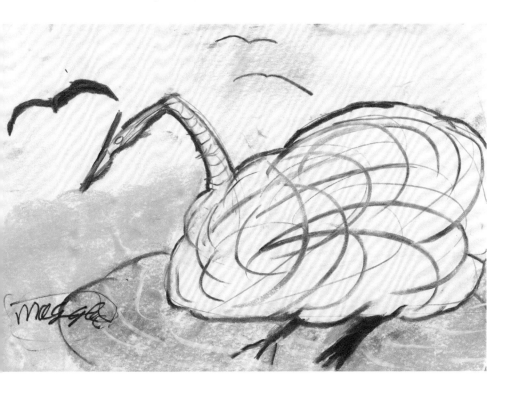

The Swan

A swan looks so elegant on the
  top, but like
    most of us in life
      it has had to paddle
    so hard to keep

          afloat.

Maggie Keppie

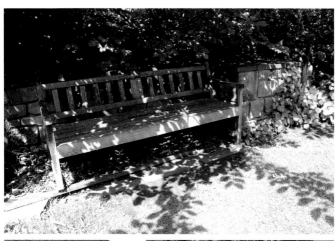

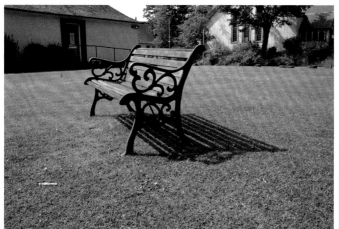

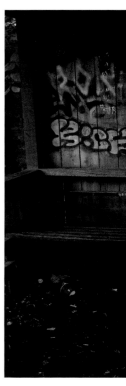

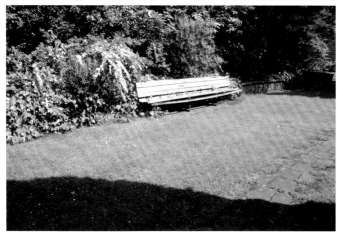

JOHN J. HARKINS

Hideouts

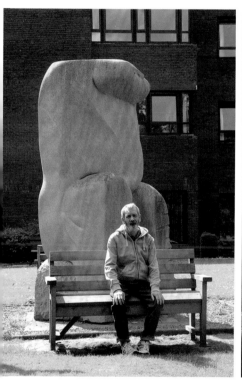 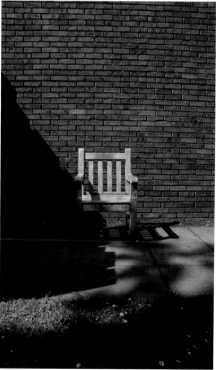

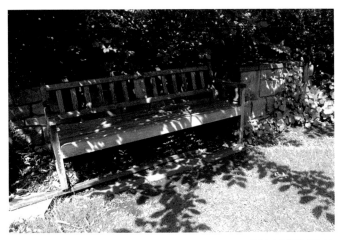

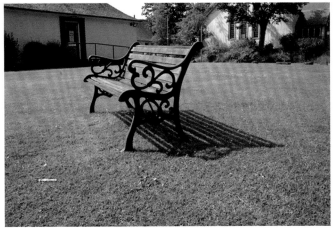

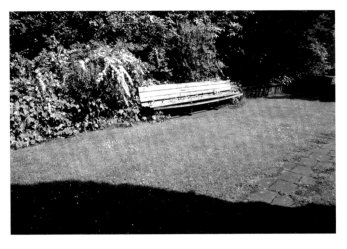

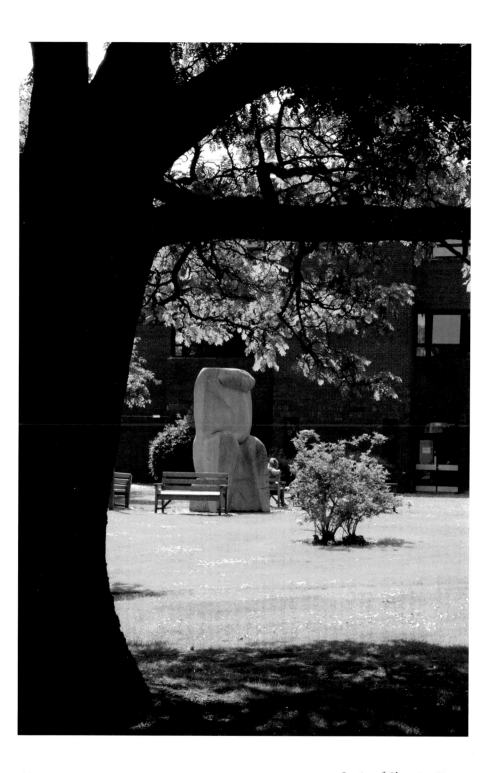

NEIL

Don't Do Drugs

After a couple of years of doing drugs I just became this totally different person.

I think it started with being at the back of the school bus, smoking cigarettes and hanging round with the cool people in school. My friend asked me if I could get LSD. I said, "I think I know a guy on the bus who could get it." It turned out to be a girl. I asked her, "Can you get LSD?"

She says, "Yeah, no problem, how many do you want?"

So I spent a couple of hours at the drug dealer's house waiting on the delivery, and then I went back to my friend's place, and we all dropped one, and we had a great time. The next weekend I thought, I'll take two this time - and I had a pretty exciting adventure. I couldn't leave the house because there was a dog on the front porch, and it wasn't my house so I didn't know what the dog was like. And from there it stemmed on to cannabis, amphetamines, cocaine – I've even used heroin.

I was obnoxious, I was nasty, I was uncaring, I was selfish, I would steal, I would lie. I got to a point in my life where I thought, I have to turn over a new leaf, I have to turn around and change things.

But at that point I became quite unwell. My mum suggested I see a psychiatrist. He diagnosed me with paranoid schizophrenia. It was quite likely that that was a result of drug use, and underlying mental health issues as well.

After about a year, having been diagnosed and using medication, I was getting into a lot of trouble with the locals – I was getting beat up for grassing, I was getting called names, they were making threats, and I tried to kill myself. Which was a very very sad day. The doctor at the hospital suggested going to Aberdeen and spending some time in the Royal Cornhill Hospital.

So I'm in in Aberdeen, I'm not using drugs, I'm not using alcohol,

I'm on medication, I'm getting therapy, really everything is going to be OK.

I moved into a hostel in Aberdeen, at the psychiatric hospital. It was a very strange place, because every day is the same.

I was always demanding a sex change operation then. On and off, I've considered an operation, to go through transition. But it just seems as though, if I put on a bra, and a nice t-shirt or whatever – "Oh he's not very well, we'll need to speak to his doctor and make sure he's ok."

I wouldn't mind wearing women's clothes. And I'm 40 now, and I'm still thinking that my boobs are going to grow. But the first time I felt that way was twenty years ago and they haven't grown. There's physical aspects to this as well as emotional.

It's a part of who I am. I'm thinking that maybe as I get older, I'll develop perhaps a little bit more determination. I find that if someone says don't do that, I won't do it.

I've always felt kind of like a woman, and a man, not at the same time usually. It's just an operation – I'll be the same person, whether I have it or not. But there's an identity that wants to come out, that wants to express itself.

I was in Aberdeen for four, maybe five years. One of the people I was living with was a very nice young lady, about the same age as myself. We got romantically involved. Then we went to Peterhead, where she's from, and we started using heroin, and alcohol, and sex, and violence. It was just ridiculous.

I decided it was time I left the girl behind, because she was a bad influence. My dad wanted me to come and live in Inverness.

So I stayed with my dad in his mobile home for a few months, and he got me a flat in the city centre. It was great – I was drug free and alcohol free. Then I thought: oh, d'you know, I fancy a bit of blow, I think I'll go and see if I can get some from somewhere. So I approached a few people in the city centre, and eventually met somebody who could get me some. I don't know who he was, but he gave me a big kiss, right on the lips!

When my friend made a joint, he would put all the hash in the joint, and we'd get sick, and we'd get up the next day and say, "Ah, I'm never doing that again." But we'd keep relapsing, so it happens a lot.

There's this guy, he's only 17 or 18, and he's into knives, and making threats. He threatened me a couple of times, and set fire to the front door when I was at my friend's house. So this boy was trouble. I thought oh god, what am I going to do? I phoned my mum and I said,

"I've got no money, I've got no house, I need to come home."

So she took me in for 6 or 7 months, back in Edinburgh. And there was heroin, and there was cocaine. And there was poor mental health, poor judgement, making silly decisions, spending money on things that I really shouldn't spend money on. There's a lot of addiction in this story.

And then I ended up in hospital here in Edinburgh, Firhill Crescent. Brilliant place to live, it was great.

When I was in the Orchard Clinic [at the REH], which must have been 2009 or 2010, one of the nurses said, "you're good with people, aren't you? You could get a voluntary job, doing stuff with people."

So I saw Angela and Katie from the [Volunteer] Hub, and we looked through some volunteer opportunities, and there was one at the hospital with the Chaplains, so I thought, why not. And before you know it I'm turning up on a Tuesday morning at Augustine's Church making tea and coffee.

At first I was like, I don't know anybody, I don't think I can remember their names, and I don't know what they're going to drink. But several weeks later, I'm like, "oh Joe, tea, milk no sugar, Katherine, coffee, milk no sugar." I kind of just took it on, and I understood that I had a position there. They make me feel good – I feel important. I even feel glamourous sometimes. If I had to leave, I think I'd miss it a lot.

Over the last six years, working with [chaplains] Maxwell and Lynn, I have a place to go, and things to do. It's just making tea and coffee, but they really appreciate it: it's part of their community, having a cup of tea and a blether. I've been a lot happier here. Now I've got things going on – I go and see my mum, make appointments on time.

I have had three relapses in the last six years – I've got a wee bit of blow, or I've got something like a legal high from the shops. But I've been drug free for a few months now. A while ago, I had a joint, on a Monday night, and texted to say "I had a joint, basically just a relapse, but I will come in tomorrow, and I hope we're busy." And we were busy, and I coped, and it was fine. I kind of like busy. I've made over 20,000 cups of tea and coffee – probably 25,000 or so now. That's a lot of tea and coffee.

Medication keeps me well. And talking - asking for help when I need it. Even if it's just over a cup of tea, a quick blether.

If I come in, and I'm maybe just a wee bit upset, Maxwell will take me aside and ask me what's going on – "you don't seem yourself".

I get delusions I'm pregnant, or that I'm going to be a millionaire. But I think a lot of people have that millionaire thing going on! Yesterday I felt, oh maybe I'm a government agent, and I'll get a Porsche and get lots of money – all these fantasies. I have those thoughts, but it's not like I act on them – it's not like I think, if I'm a spy then I can steal that, and it'll be fine. It's nothing like a James Bond film at all. It's more like, "Hello Crimestoppers, I think there's a dealer next door to me"!

I don't know what happens to those thoughts now, I think I just put them away, and get on with my day – do my usual things. Maybe tomorrow I'll think about it again, but it's no big deal.

I think doing my voluntary work – making my teas and coffees and being nice to people, being around people – that helps.

I have an action plan, WRAP, so now if I have a problem, I identify the problem, I think about some logical application I can make to it, and the whole problem goes away, and I'm OK.

I get support from Richmond Fellowship. They provide me with an hour every evening during the week, and at the weekend I get between five and six hours in the afternoon. We went to St Andrews on the bus for a trip, and we've been to Aberdeen, and we'll get the tram to the Gyle Centre, do a bit of shopping. We have a great time, and they're great people to work with.

I think it's important to have company, even if it is from support workers. We'll go to a coffee shop, have a coffee and a cake and some blether. I see them as mates – not mates like "let's go to the pub" or anything silly, we're not going to cross any lines – boundaries are important. It's just good company, and I do like them very much. We get on famously.

I just thank God for all the great stuff that's going on. Because without Him, and my support workers, I'd probably be in quite a bad place. Because when you get mixed up with drugs, the kind of people that you meet, they're not always nice.

There aren't many bad things that are happening in my life now; there aren't many people who don't like me. So I'm dead grateful for everything I've got that's good.

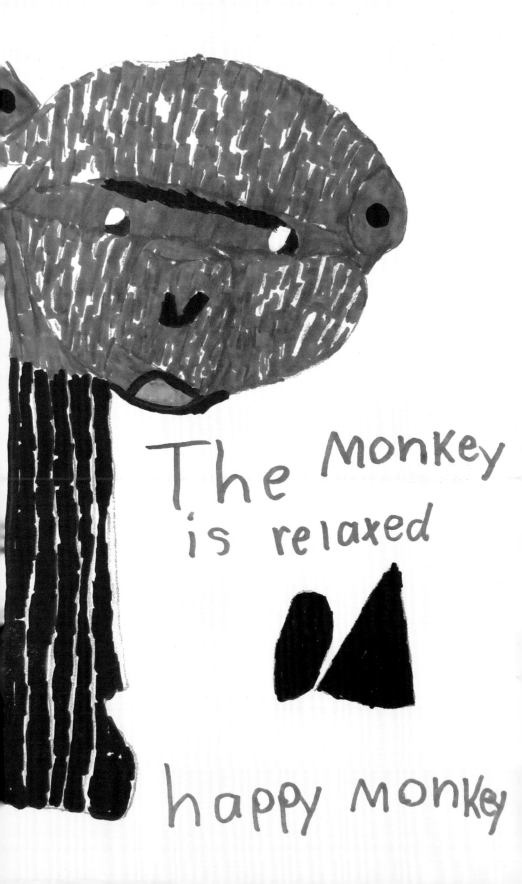

The Monkey
is relaxed

happy Monkey

ANGELA FARR
KATIE SMITH

Kindness and purpose: volunteering at the Royal Edinburgh

Tell us a bit about your jobs, and the Volunteer Hub.

Katie: The aim of the Volunteer Hub is to do everything we can to promote recovery and well-being in the hospital through the use of volunteers. We do that partially by bringing in members of the public who want to volunteer, and partially by promoting volunteering to patients.

Patients get involved in all sorts of different activities. A lot of that is in the hospital, if people aren't well enough to be heading out, but we aim to build people up to volunteer in the community.

Then we also have members of the public – people who want to work in the NHS who want to get experience, some retired people, some people from the local area who want to help out.

> *We buddy people up, so that we can provide that extra support for patients to be doing things that they find joy in.*

Angela: The unique thing that we do is that we involve patients in volunteering in the hospital, which isn't done to our knowledge anywhere else.

Katie: We try to use the patient volunteering programme to make the hospital a nicer place, with the additional benefit that it helps people feel that they're contributing to their community.

Can you tell me a few of the roles that patients might have?

Angela: We meet the person first, and then we try to find out what their strengths and their interests are, and then we build something around that. Some people can do ten minutes a week, some people do three, four hours a week, and it really depends on what people's motivation for volunteering is. Is it about getting up and out of bed, or is it about getting a job, or is it about the activity? What is it that would get someone ticking? If someone comes with an idea, we either try and create it or we will approach other staff that help us support that.

We've people working on the fruit and veg stall, a lot of plant care, admin work… Somebody who was on the acute admissions ward for quite a long time volunteered with us two mornings a week, and set up an Excel spreadsheet that none of us could do.

A lot of patients are involved in different volunteering tasks in the library, which we run: it might be around books, but it might also be about supporting groups that are going on.

Katie: So there are jobs that can suit everybody, and part of the creativity of our job is trying to find the thing that works for people, and trying to find how someone's skills can benefit the hospital community, which is very rewarding when you find it.

So we see it as quite vital that we create the right ethos in people – treating people kindly, respectfully, as people that have got something to offer.

What do you think helps people to get well and stay well?

Katie: Kindness, and time, and listening to people. Meaningful activity – it has to be something that is important to that person and is the right thing for them.

Angela: The thing that [public volunteers] can offer is it is that experience of being with people that are not clinical staff, or people that are paid to be with you, which is really important. We can influence people who come into this type of work at the very beginning of this journey.

It is really good for people to have people in the hospital that don't know about the difficult times and the problems. It is so important that there is that opportunity for people to put forward the sense of themselves that isn't "I'm a patient" or "I'm unwell".

that moment of crisis. It is about, "I'm interested in Ancient Egypt and I used to live in India" – whatever it is that is important to that person.

Angela: In a hospital setting, I think there are a lot of opportunities for patients to engage in, but sometimes it is about the levels of support to enable that to happen – to get off the ward. I think it can be a barrier.

Katie: If people aren't getting good human connection, that's a real hindrance. Of course within this setting, there are a lot of conflicting demands for people's time and it is easy, I think, for people to not get the time that they really need, and the kindness that they really need.

It is a difficult setting to work in, and it is a difficult setting for patients to be in – so anything that we can do to give people that more peaceful time is great.

What is working in the hospital like as a Third Sector organisation?

Angela: I think we're in a really privileged position because all our interactions are around positive things – we're not having to have conversations about medication or restriction, we're there just to make things a little bit nicer for people. And I feel that is really valued within the hospital.

Katie: There is so much support in risk assessment. We're able to involve people from the Orchard clinic with very serious convictions, we're able to do volunteering with people because of the hospital setting and the clinical team's oversight of that. It is much more challenging in the community, and if you don't have that partnership.

Angela: I suppose the main issue for us, like most Third Sector organisations, is the year on year funding. The really lucky thing for us in relation to our funders, is that they have always been very supportive around what we do and how we do it, so we've been able to be really responsive to what is needed.

What are your thoughts on the new hospital?

Katie: It is really nice to see an opportunity for more privacy for the patients. I hope that the wards will be a less stressful environment, because they've got their own space.

Angela: And their own access to green space – that hit me, that you can actually see green space from every bedroom – I think that is quite important. This hospital does have a very strong sense of community, compared to other ones I've worked in – so the challenge is that that sense of community is kept when it's split, and when it is in a much more clinical-looking environment.

We've been here ten years now, and we've always been incredibly supported, particularly by the OT [occupational therapy] staff. We have the same idea about ways of working with people, so that has been a really natural fit for us.

Katie: And lots more patients coming in future as well – the finished site will be much bigger, so it is a bit harder to hold onto that.

Angela: People like ourselves and the Hive are going to be a long way from the new hospital, so that is a concern – how that will impact on our services, because there isn't a space in the new hospital for us.

Katie: I think it will be a few years of constant change, with the building works. I hope as much as possible the trees and the green environment stays. I think it will be sad to see some of that turn into a building site.

What are your hopes and dreams for the Volunteer Hub?

Angela: That we long continue, and that we get more embedded, and that our impact for patients is greater as the years go by and that they have more opportunities to be involved with us.

Katie: We're always incredibly busy, so to feel like we were able to give everybody the opportunities that they're looking for and to be able to get to know people and find tailor-made volunteering activities for people – just doing more of what we're doing.

Angela: And because we work in the third sector we have to say this: we would like stable funding.

Katie: And a smooth move around the next few years of building works.

What is the most important lesson that your job has taught you?

Katie: For me, it is that you should always make the effort to be kind to people and to take the time for people. It is always more important than answering the phone or looking at the emails or all these other demands. Be kind always.

Angela: It is appreciating the small things and not looking for, "everyone is going to be out volunteering in the community", because that is not realistic, but knowing people are doing something in the moment and that is good.

Katie: I see other people that I know getting incredibly stressed at work, and see other people's work impacting on their mental health, and I think the thing about working here is that you realise how important your own mental health is and how vulnerable you are. So that idea that we could all be in this situation, and that you do things to make sure that you look after yourself, and that your wellbeing is important.

> *It doesn't matter what crisis people are going through, or how desperate people are, there is an innate something in everyone – that people want to help others. So if you can tap into that at the right time, then it is very powerful.*

Reliever of st

"*Art is an excellent therapy for your mental health wellbeing. It keeps me focused and it makes me happy.*"

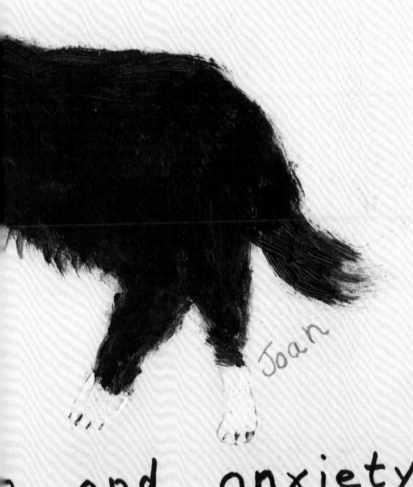

Joan

s and anxiety

Joan Templeton, *Shep*

TONY CHAN

New Beginnings

We've been through the good times, we've been through the bad times

Together we can face a brighter future

Concentrate on the positive, have faith for the future, hope for the best

and expect the best in life, work towards it, there's a lot to do, no time for a rest

You are stronger than you know, your light shines brightly – the goodness in you, it shows

You bring meaning and purpose in people's lives, as you lessen their strife

You are sunshine after the rain, there's nothing about you that's plain

A smile from you brightens up the darkest places, it's what you want from people's faces

You have a gift of listening, with compassion you are glistening

Your gifts and talents make you stand out and show, makes you happy and glow

Your sense of humour brings laughter and a giggle to all

You can make a difference, to someone else, because it is your call

Surely you are special and unique, you are a treasure, you are certainly not weak

You definitely live up to your name, as you will never be ashamed

Of the day you were born, the cord can never be broken, never be torn

Life would be a lot duller and bleak without your presence

Your spirit and soul shine out, from your very essence

Make the most of your life and serve others

Because at the end of the day we are all sisters and brothers

People Make Change

Some of the many individuals involved in the Royal Edinburgh Hospital talk about changes they have witnessed and people who have helped make them happen. Eight individual interviews, and one group interview were carried out. Excerpts are brought together here, as if they are all talking together in the same room.

THE BUILDING

Interviewer: Have you seen changes at the Royal Edinburgh Hospital?

Tim Montgomery: So, you'll be aware that the site is over 200 years old. This building we're sitting in is 160 years old. When I came here others had been trying to rebuild the hospital for – at that point it would have been 20 years. There wasn't really a strong belief that it would ever happen, but we're now a week away from moving into the first phase of the brand-new hospital.

Maggie McIvor: I can still remember picking everybody up to get involved again, they had put so much effort and so much time into the planning for that hospital and everybody was thinking there isn't any point because it's never going to happen. Now it's happening, so it's wonderful.

Patricia Whalley: I mean, even going back to when initially we were thinking of building the new Royal Edinburgh, they were going to take it to Little France, and there was a big uprising in Edinburgh and the Lothians to say, "Please no!" and we all fought very, very hard. I don't know if it was Dave Budd [Patients Council, Project Manager] or I don't know if it was because the Patients Council kept on about it, but it was reversed. We like to feel that the whole of Edinburgh, through the service users and the consultations, got it.

Tim Davidson: I was disappointed that the plans that we were talking about in the mid-1980s hadn't come to fruition. I must pay tribute to the people in Lothian: before I arrived there had been a lot of work already done. In my first year or two, I worked with colleagues to put some priority into generating the master plan for the entire site, which you'll know is a really ambitious and extensive programme for redeveloping not just the mental health services on that site, but also learning disability services, and also rehabilitation services.

Maggie McIvor: I believe that the new hospital is actually getting built because Patricia encountered Geoff Huggins [then Head of Mental Health, Scottish Government] in a meeting, who at that point was head of the mental health unit for the Scottish Government. She asked him when the new hospital was going to be built. And he said "Oh I thought it had. Those papers passed over my desk ages ago." And the next day, he came to visit the hospital and then things actually happened.

Interviewer: Can I ask, are the patients themselves active in the development?

Dick Fitzpatrick: In the early days, I put a paper together for the project board that asked that when we do anything in relation to design or option appraisal, there needed to be the same number of service users as there are other professionals or other organisations represented round the table. In other words, 50% service user involvement. The board agreed and we have achieved it at every stage. I think it's reasonable to say that service users have had a very significant input to the Royal Ed. Their fingerprints are all over it. And I've actually seen that come through in the design itself.

Maggie McIvor: Our feeling right through the process was that the design team were really listening. Dick, who was the project manager for phase one for many years, he really moved mountains to get the process started.

Dick Fitzpatrick: It's not all down to me. Everybody was behind it and that's what made it work.

Linda Irvine: It was about four years ago, we created a public social partnership called Green Space Art Space. We invited patients, staff, members of the public, carers and people with relatives or friends who had been admitted to the Royal Edinburgh. There was probably over a hundred of us in the room. There was so much synergy between what everybody said and there were lots of ambitious ideas. Everybody wanted to feel safe and secure, people wanted to feel that there was a therapeutic value in the green space, and that we were nurturing the environment.

ATTITUDES

Martin McAlpine: The building, yes, but it's the people and the work they do. Changing attitudes is fundamental, much more important than the bricks and mortar.

Linda Irvine: There have been pretty significant changes in people's attitudes. One of the first things I did was to arrange an event with people who use services and staff. But I'm really embarrassed to say that we actually had separate tables for service users. Because service users and staff didn't feel comfortable about sitting together.

Interviewer: Oh dear.

Linda Irvine: I know! If you think about now, we just did Taking Stock last week, which is our annual conference, everybody just sits together. People just come as themselves. And they can choose to have conversations or not, about what their background is, or what their experiences are.

Tim Davidson: There's been a general shift in public opinion, and in professional opinion about mental illness. There have been so many people involved in that. Some of it is societal, over decades.

Patients Council volunteer: I've also had a real feeling that the new building is going to go alongside some new attitudes and some new doings. So, it's still too early to say what will happen. Whether the old buildings will also be kept, with the older statues, having a new building goes together with having new times, a new generation and new ways of doing things altogether.

SERVICES

Elizabeth Gallagher: When I first came, my feeling was it was very custodial, it was very rule-orientated. It was very hard to push through any kind of change. Being able to say, "well actually I don't mind taking the medication to the bed, because they've just gone to bed at six o'clock this morning, and to pull them back out of bed now just to come up here doesn't make sense to me," was a change. So, there was a bit of gentle persuasion went on. But if you were to compare then and now, it's chalk and cheese.

Michele Harrison: I always wanted a revolution, but actually change is an evolutionary process.

Tim Davidson: The mid-1980s was an exciting time because it was at the beginning of the development of community based mental health services.

Michele Harrison: I was at a meeting with support and accommodation providers and a representative from housing suggested we submit a paper to the board who agree housing priorities. The paper was submitted in January and priorities were changed in April, enabling people to move into living options that work for them and create supported places for people to move out of hospital quicker. Three people are moving out as a result.

Lesley Smith: I found myself getting more involved in recovery work as this spoke more to my heart and my mind, and there was energy about it! Delivering training through the Lothian Recovery Network was empowering as it was co-produced and I was able to influence the way NHS services were being delivered. Seeing myself as a trainer, rather than a patient or service user, allowed me to engage with people in a different way, which was more mutual. It also meant I was tapping into my goals in life before I became unwell, reignited my energy and it all contributed to where I am today.

Alison Robertson: I used to give talks to student nurses at Edinburgh Napier University about what it's like to be a service user, and I think it gives them a different idea of what it's like to be ill, and that recovery is possible. I talk about being suicidal right up until – well, you can see my recovery now. So, it's about the nurses having hope as well, that people can get better. You hope to encourage them, and tell them that any kindness that they do, that they might not see it blossom the next day, but in time.

PEOPLE

Linda Irvine: There are always key people from the service user community, and from the staff community, who really encourage change, and can be quite inspiring.

Elizabeth Gallagher: I don't know if you want actual names, there's quite a list of them. Donna McComish, would be one [Charge Nurse] and Trevor Jones [Charge Nurse] – both have dedicated their entire careers to making significant changes in this type of service. Derek Chiswick, consultant psychiatrist, who has retired now. Colin

Mackintosh [Charge Nurse] has retired now, and Andy Notman [Charge Nurse].

Martin McAlpine: Could I throw in a word for the mental health chaplains? The Department of Spiritual Care. It used to be called the Chaplaincy Department, but that was restricted just to Christians. So, they broadened it and it's now the Department of Spiritual Care, and they've been advocating the patients voice.

Tim Montgomery: It does feel like we've had a lot more involvement in other providers' ways of working, and that has opened a lot of people's eyes – like the Volunteer Centre, Cyrenians, SAMH, The Hive, Artlink and working with some of the clinical staff. OTs [occupational therapists] quite often are leading lights.

Linda Irvine: The Patients Council have become really skilled at saying what they're thinking. They have their own meetings so that they know that they're representing groups of people rather than just individual viewpoints. When I first started I don't think people were really aware of what collective advocacy was. It's much more visible now.

Simon Porter: I can only say how he changed me, but but Albert Nicolson [Patient's Council] taught me how to do activism and survive it emotionally. He's been an activist since the 60s, I think.

Alison Robertson: Albert helps a lot of people and quietly. He talks about how he found his own recovery and give up medication. He gives people hope.

Simon Porter: I just want to mention two more people, Alison Prosser and Ronnie Jack, because they're not here anymore. They were involved in the art side of advocacy. They both died in the last year, and Shirley too, she was influential in terms of older people's services.

Interviewer: Lastly Elizabeth, any ideas on how people might influence change in the future?

Elizabeth Gallagher: Well, I'm very conscious that I retire at the end of the year. The people that I mentioned earlier, we're all of the same age. So, in the space of a few years you're losing all the historical knowledge that we have in our heads. Our recent focus has been around contingency planning, and how we make sure that everything done thus far doesn't get undone. Which I know sounds slightly arrogant, but it's not meant to be. We're working to make sure that people coming into the service understand how and why we do things the way we do. Albeit, we're always open to good ideas and we'll say that to people. "We can learn from you coming in. Don't be sitting thinking - I'd better not say." We want to know.

Interviewees:

Tim Montgomery: Services Director, Royal Edinburgh Hospital

Maggie McIvor: Development Worker, Patients Council

Patricia Whalley: Chair, Patients Council

Tim Davidson: Chief Executive, NHS Lothian

Dick Fitzpatrick: Project Manager, NHS Lothian

Linda Irvine: Strategic Programme Manager, Mental Health and Wellbeing, NHS Lothian

Martin McAlpine: Volunteer, Patients Council

Elizabeth Gallagher: Clinical Nurse Manager, Royal Edinburgh Hospital

Michele Harrison: Research Fellow, Wayfinder Partnership, Queen Margaret University

Lesley Smith: Network Officer, Scottish Recovery Network

Alison Robertson: Vice Chair, Patients Council

Simon Porter: Coordinator, Patients Council

Interviewers – CAPS Independent Advocacy Volunteers & Staff: Shirley-Anne Collie, Marianne Mackintosh, Theresa Trotter, Pam van de Brug, Jane Crawford & Victoria Jackson

A NON

Horrible moments to home comforts

What's your history with the hospital?
I was an outpatient from '94 'til 2008/9 when I became an inpatient. The first was six weeks and then I was let out. It didn't work out, so I was taken back in.

What was it that led up to you being an outpatient?
I was divorced and my parents died. I moved house to Shetland, where I was diagnosed as needing to go to the Aberdeen mental hospital. I was only six weeks there. I got back to Shetland and decided to come south again. The doctors up there referred me to the outpatients' clinic here.

Was that helpful?
Not really.

What kept you well during that time? What was it that helped, if anything?
If anything, quite. There was Stepping Stones; that was a mental health facility, arts facility, writing and painting and stained-glass work and lots of things. It's run by the university's outreach. Unfortunately, that went bust, so Stepping Stones had to close.

How long were you an inpatient for?
A year. I was diagnosed with schizophrenic psychosis.
Katie: Well, I guess it's similar things in reverse – low expectations of people.
The public volunteers have never seen the people they work with in

What was it like to be in hospital at that time?
Horrible. It was very scruffy and very much in need of being done up. The washing machine didn't work properly and our belongings were put in black bags under the stairs. It was grotty.

What led up to you being admitted?
I was having hallucinations through walls and seeing people in the street. I lived off the High Street, which is very busy. The police were involved with me.

Was there anything in the hospital that helped you to get well, if anything?
I think my medication and the activities nurse.

What kind of activities did you do?
We went to Cramond and had a cup of tea, which was nice. There were various meetings on the ward to discuss the papers.

How were they helpful for you?
Their kindness showed through. They also had the OT assistant to see me and we went out for coffee. Such a nice woman.

Was there anything in the hospital that was unhelpful? You said a little bit about it being scruffy and not a very nice environment. Was there anything else?
The way the staff treated me. They flirted with me. They were known flirts. It was most unhelpful. That's putting it nicely.

Is there anything you wish someone had told you when you came to the hospital?

That it would be very stressful. I can remember I didn't have much space of my own and what I did have was taken away from me. One night at about 11 o'clock they came and said, "We are putting you in another room." They were not nice things that happened. It isn't a bed of roses in the hospital. We thought we were hallucinating through walls and singing a wee song about polonium 90. We were all very worried about the railway carrying polonium 90.

How was it being around lots of other people who were also having difficulties?
I had to be very careful. Not to offend people and not to get involved in their troubles. I think it will be much better when the new hospital is built and opened, when people have their own rooms.

What advice would you give to someone who is being admitted to hospital?
Try and be as quiet as possible. They might be raving or having hallucinations, but the staff would see that and dose you up accordingly. They'll fit in easier because it's really a little community, the ward.

What was it like to be discharged?
I was pleased to be going into my new accommodation, but I felt a bit lonely, shall we say. It soon passed away, that feeling. They were so good to me. They sorted my money. They got a dentist, got a doctor, all the things that are necessary for good living.

What kind of accommodation do you live in now? Is it supported?
Yes. It's a little flat.

Is it a good space to be in?
Absolutely marvellous.

What's good about it?
The way the staff treat people with dignity.

What do you think helps you to be well just now? What helps you to stay well?
My activities, like the support agency's reference group, which is a group that meets once every six weeks to discuss things the big board haven't the space to discuss.

What kind of things do you discuss?
How to involve more people... Oh, quite a lot of things.

What do you get out of being part of the reference group? How does it make you feel to be part of that?
Marvellous. I enjoy it very much. It's run by a dear lady.

You get on well with her?
Extremely well, yes. The same sort of thing for my housing provider.

So you're on the reference group for them as well?
Scrutiny group.

Can you tell me a bit more about the purpose of the groups?
To give the tenants a say in how the organisation is run. There's the scrutiny group and there's the tenants' association, which are different. You have to be elected onto the tenants' association, and I'm seeing if I can get elected onto it at this moment.

What makes you want to be a part of it? What is it that appeals about it?
I always like to be in the know.

So you're actually quite busy with different things around your housing.
Yes, and I go to a writing group.

What kind of things do you write?
We've been writing about structures recently – bridges and roads.

How long have you been doing that for?
Years and years.

What do you think you get out of writing?
I'm learning to express myself, because I've been a very shut-away person.

What's that like, to be bringing things out there a bit more?
Good.

Do you feel like it affects the rest of your life?
The only way to put it, it makes me more understanding of other people's troubles, being part of that group.

Are there any other things that you're involved in?
The Scottish Mental Health Arts and Film Festival. I'm on the St. Augustine drop-in.

So you're helping with that group's involvement with the arts and film festival?
It will be writing up the stories of the drop-in.

Have you been going to the drop-in for a long time?
Many years.

What do you get from it?
Company, and knowing what's the matter with other people, how one can help.

What do you think is the most important lesson that life has taught you?

To reach out to people who can help, because I've always been a very shut-away person.

What are your hopes and dreams for the future?
I try and live day by day. I've been taught that, as one isn't that well sometimes. To be helpful to the organisations I'm part of because they're very, very nice.

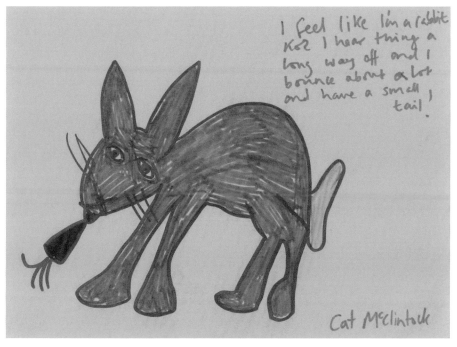

I feel like I'm a rabbit koz I hear thing a long way off and I bounce about a lot and have a small tail!

Cat McClintock

Cat McClintock, *Rabbit*

ANNE-LOUISE LOWREY

Home

I had been awarded a furnished tenancy with the council. The flat was painted and carpeted, with a bed, a wardrobe, a cooker, a fridge and a three-piece suite. It was so exciting to have the basics of a home all to myself. My family were very pleased and so was I, but still deep inside I was insecure. Yet another episode and admittance to hospital meant that I was definitely going to have to have injections of antipsychotics for the rest of my life.

There was a tug of war within me - one wanting to do it and carry on living - and another that kept planning my suicide, even though there were good things in my life.

The injection made me feel ill and bloated. I was sleeping 15 hours a night and apathetic about everything. I felt so insignificant, and tried hard to blend into the background wherever I went, but that wasn't to be. People seemed to notice fault with me – often about the way I looked and how low my motivation for everything was.

One person who criticised me a lot was one of my flatmates at the time. He would often tell me I was fat and plain, as well as weak of character and dependant, as if I didn't have a lot going for me. Comments like; "you look hefty in that dress Anne-Louise" or "could you ever imagine yourself being good looking?"

I didn't have a lot of confidence anyway, so this type of treatment just reinforced my belief that I was rubbish and worthless. I wasn't even worth giving a token compliment to. The thing that cemented this was, one day, I was upstairs on a bus (trying to blend into the background), when a young guy started to mock me, "My God, what a baby you are!" Before long his friends joined in and they all shouted 'rover' at me over and over again, calling me a dog. As I got up to leave, it felt like the whole bus was shouting at me.

A couple of similar incidents like this led me to the conclusion that it was the medication that made me stand out so much and look so vulnerable. I always gained weight when I took it and it affected the way I walked. My skin was drained of natural colour, and a frugal diet, along with profuse cigarette smoking, seemed to cause blotches and spots on top of this. At a time when I had very low self-esteem, the medication felt like a hindrance rather than a solution. I had stopped it twice before, and both times had to be admitted to hospital for long periods until I got back on an even keel (or relative sanity).

Nonetheless, I was taking the medication, confused about the future and depressed about how ugly and stupid and untalented and ungifted I believed I was. Even things I had used to do like arts and crafts, I just couldn't seem to do any more. If I thought it couldn't get any worse, I was sitting up late in the flat one night, about a couple of weeks before I was to move when the phone rang. It was my sister, crying, saying that something had happened to our brother. It turned out he had been sitting on the windowsill of his bedsit at the end of the night, when he slipped and fell. He was killed instantly.

Our whole family was thrown into turmoil and grief. Witnessing my parents' sorrow was almost more than I could bear. Of course we all felt it very deeply, as did cousins and friends, other relatives and colleagues. There was a huge coming together of souls to honour this young life that had been lost. It somehow felt like a sacrifice.

As with all tragedies, some hope always shines through, and for me it was the fact that I forgot about myself and the nasty things people had said and done to me. I was grateful just to be alive. The opinion of a lads' night out wasn't important compared with what had happened. I have always felt guilty that it took something as devastating as this to make me strong. Of course, it's not that I didn't know that this type of bullying was done by shallow, people. It was just that I was hurt and upset and embarrassed regardless and even now, I still find it difficult to say that "names will never hurt me."

Soon after the funeral, I moved into my new home. It was near my parents' house and in those days they could easily walk it. They visited me shell shocked and grieving. I felt the need to comfort them somehow. Through the natural course of the conversation we got onto discussing the medication. My mum simply asked me to comply with it as they couldn't go through any more heartache. I agreed, and even though I didn't feel very sure, I remembered a woman called 'D' that I had met in hospital and her words of wisdom: "If you can't do it for yourself, then do it for somebody else!"

I was able to apply this, and within a couple years of taking it continually, my body seemed to settle down and I wasn't so zonked. I am now sitting in the same living room, 26 years later, with the candles burning and many little mementos of my time spent here. It has proven to be a haven for me in good times and bad – and I am still on the medication. 22 years ago, I had an admittance to the Royal Edinburgh Hospital, but have had none since – thanks to the medication – and a lot of great people that have been, and are, in my life. Yes, it does have side effects and it is bad for your body – but so does being continually in and out of hospital. I feel as though I am very lucky and really didn't expect to even live this long. But I'm 51 years old and I have a partner of 18 years. We don't live together, but do love each other.

I'm not rich or outwardly successful, but I have a few things going for me – one of them being my life! And yes I am afraid of the Government, DWP, Brexit and the general problems of the world. But I will always remember 'D' – a fellow patient: "If you can't do it for yourself, then do it for somebody else!" When it's applied to things you want to do anyway, like stopping smoking or taking exercise it can really give you motivation to think of somebody else who wants you to do that too.

Recipe for a melting moment

Anne-Louise Lowrey

Take several drops of rain
And a pint of sunshine
Toss them onto a wet balcony
And sauté
Making sure that you remember
To add a spoonful
Of spider's web

Stir well until it turns a golden colour
And leave to settle

Then take a large bowl
Of mother earth
Add a handful of laughter seeds
While a plump pigeon is cooing
In the background among the weeds

Next, blend all the ingredients together
Into a compassionate heart
Finely chop a good bunch of unconditional love
And whisk to create a melting moment

Sublime!

MARIANNE MACKINTOSH

Near and Far

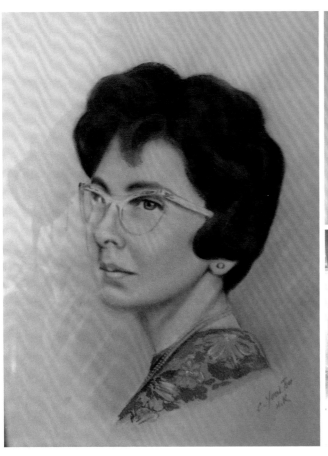

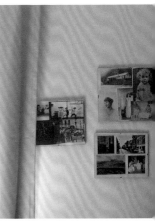

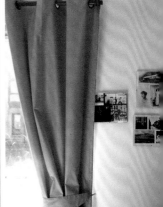

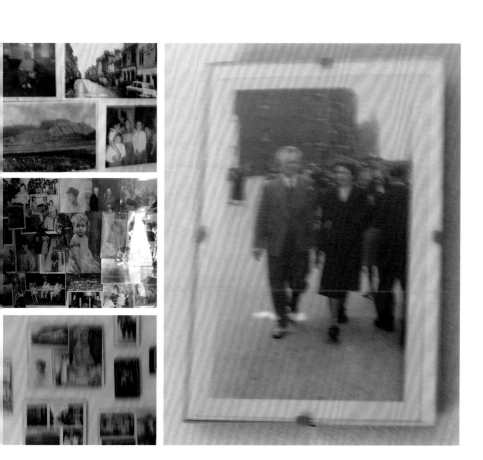

ESTHER

Keys

Coming to Firrhill was life changing for me in a very, very, good way. It made me start to see the real world through my own eyes and not through nurses' eyes.

I'm not living by lock and key now either; I've got my own lock and key which I carry round my round my neck 24/7 so it can remind me never to go back to where I was in a Hospital Locked Ward.

It is good to have a room here in Firrhill. I have my own orthopaedic bed, plasma TV, sofa, rug and chair. I chose everything apart from the orthopaedic bed myself.

My advice to others in hospital now is – Keep positive, don't look backwards, always look ahead. There is a chance for you. I was there and thought I'd never break free, but I did.

Now I'm just looking forward to getting a little house somewhere and getting my family all together for a meal in my home. I'm just waiting on the right place.

When I move on, I'll be happy that someone else will appreciate and enjoy living at Firrhill. They can keep the room neat and tidy - or how they like it – as long as it is comfy and suits and pleases them.

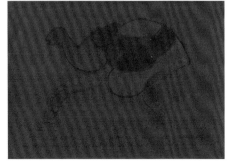

Karina Davies, Turtle

"Mental health recovery is a long slow process, but it can be achieved with the right support."

CLAIRE MARTIN

From the Heart

I have worked as a specialist occupational therapist within the *Progressing on Both Fronts Project* – a partnership trying out new models of care to support people to live in the community – since April 2016. The Project supports people residing both at Myreside Ward in the Hospital and living in their own flats at the Firrhill Residence. The most rewarding aspect of my job is working with people, whether that is in a one-to-one or group setting. I enjoy getting to know each person and finding out how they wish to be supported to improve their health and well being. We then tailor our support to each individual through a combined support plan that details what goals the person has for the future and how they wish to be assisted to reach those goals. This helps ensure that all the partner agencies supporting the person work together.

During the last year I have been delighted to see people get closer to living the lives they wish to lead. Some people have increased their physical fitness through walking more or taking up swimming or cycling again. Others have found new meaningful occupations such as having their own allotments to grow vegetables or undertaking new volunteer work roles of working in a library, a garden or local shops. It has been great to see people doing daily activities more independently, whether it is learning to cook an omelette or going shopping themselves. We've all worked together to improve the living environments for those residing at Firrhill and Myreside. People have been involved in creating artworks to make their living areas more homely and in deciding what flowers and vegetables we will plant in their garden areas to make their outdoor living spaces more pleasant.

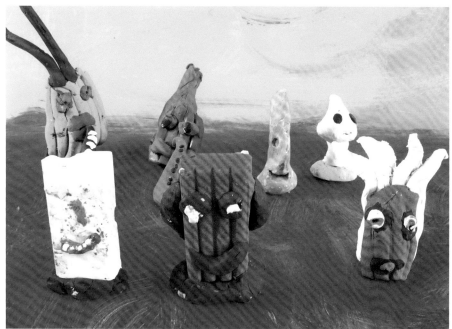

Daz T, Wee Dudes

CAROL GRAHAM

The Road to Crazy Paving

So I start again. Writing my book; the one nobody really sees. The one dripping with drama; the one full of humour and the human condition. What I like most is to analyse other people – and I'm at a good angle. As a disabled woman, it gives me a chance to find out if others accept me as normal.

The thing is, how do you define the normal? I see it as a family: the mother, the father and the 2.5 children all sitting down for breakfast, teasing each other and occasionally giving tidbits to the dog. Does that image really exist? I've written about it for years. I've never fitted into the 'normal' category, for which I am eternally grateful. Christmas has come and gone. That's the one time of year that families and what goes with them rears their ugly heads.

There's lots to write about as I think a little deeper. My job, the life I had after leaving my job. And the life before. I see before me snippets of my life as a child, as a teenager, as an adult. I never believed I'd live to adulthood. Being a child was hard enough. I was always being bossed by my parents, my teachers, other kids.

And it doesn't seem to change after hitting adulthood. I'm disabled. Therefore I need help. I'm vulnerable. Treat me with kid gloves. Talk to me as if I had a hearing problem. Look at me and think "Thank God, it's her and not me." Then I think I'm too sensitive. Where's your sense of humour. Maybe I should diversify. Use my writing skills in other ways. Little stories, small perceptions in life like growing up in small Canadian town on the shores of Lake Ontario. "For the newly-wed and the nearly-dead": a quote from a friend of my father. 'Little Chicago', someone called it. Yes, there was always a crime wave going on. Oh, the talk in town. "What next? Our children aren't safe."

I hated small-town life. It was so small. Everyone knew everyone's movements.

"You're not lonely," – my mother. "Neither am I. I've lots of friends."

"Do you think Dad's lonely? He's away three weeks out of four and he spends time in hotels. What does he do on the road?"

"How should I know? We're happy being at home together, aren't we? We can relax, have our meals in front of the TV, chat."

"Yeah, but we're not the normal family."

"My family in Scotland weren't normal either. Look, I like the TV. When the man asks 'do you know where your children are?' Thanks to crime, he's in cell block 11, in Sing Sing."

"I should read more. Dad's a great reader."

"We always do the *Globe and Mail* Crossword every Sunday. It's good for the brain."

"What will become of me? Will I get a job? Will I get married?"

"What makes you think I can look into the future and predict your fate?"

"Why did you marry Dad?"

"He was good-looking and his feet didn't smell."

"Is that it? You're spending the rest of your life with someone and that's the reason you married?"

"You always have to probe, Carol, to analyse. Why don't you take life as it comes?"

"I guess it's because I've never fitted in. I don't have brothers and sisters."

It doesn't pay to feel sorry for yourself. No one really wants to know. I have no family. They all died within five years of each other. Falling down like a pack of cards. I can look back and laugh at the situations I got into with my family.

My Dad was away a lot. Mother said he was 'on the road'. In my mind I visualise a strip of highway with hotels and bars and shops on either side. A time for excitement and new experiences. That wasn't the reality. Dad was staying in hotels meeting people occasionally, and yes, drinking. Like everything else in his life, what he did on the road remained a mystery.

I once read Arthur Miller's autobiography. I wanted to know his relationship with Marilyn Monroe. She was a hero of mine. Vulnerable, lonely, used, her affairs were renowned. But I really wanted to know about Arthur Miller's book, *Death of a Salesman*. Was that Dad's story? Away from family life. A single man. Who did he meet? Did he get involved with other people 'on the road'? These are the questions I still ask myself, and there's no one to answer them.

Come on, Carol, don't get maudlin. Life is what you make. Kick off your shoes, have a fag, and enjoy. Every day is different.

"I'm bored. I wish the holidays were over!" I moaned.

"Back to school. New friends, new things to learn," said Mother.

"UGH! I hate school. It's boring. All the teachers are on the verge of nervous breakdowns."

"All of them?"

"Only the semi-bright ones. Does it take brains to have a nervous breakdown?"

"Such talk! Stop it. You're just having growning pains!"

"Growing pains? You mean periods, larger breasts?"

"Don't bring that up again. So I thought you had cancer."

"And the doctor said, 'Haven't you heard of development, Mrs. Graham?' So embarassing!"

"How do you think I felt?"

"I like your stories of the war. You make it sound so much fun."

"It was!"

"Was Alloa involved in the war?"

"Yes. A bomb dropped and killed a cow. And something happened in Fishcross. A man was drinking his soup at the kitchen table and something large and silver shot down through the roof. It was a bomb. The local papers interviewed him. 'I was just drinking my soup. And was interrupted by this big, silver thing.' 'What did you do?' 'I finished my soup.' No-one panics in Fishcross."

Remember the shy little girl in the Prime of Miss Jean Brodie? She had a stutter. "She tells l-lovely stories." So did my mother. Funny, lovely stories. Was everyone in Alloa a character? Mother said that when she was young, she'd go downtown with a friend and pretend she was blind.

"Mother, that's terrible."

"I know. I shouldn't have told you."

Bou Bou Synnar

Hell-in-a-cell

robertbrownboubou@gmail.com

What's your history with the hospital?
When I was thirteen years old, my mum told me I was raped by
my grandad when I was three. I started hearing voices, and I saw a
psychiatrist for two years. The voices told me to call women 'bitches' as
they walked past me. It took me two years to overcome this.

The first time I ever got admitted was in April 1995, when I was
25 years old. I got kicked out of a cult in Leeds. I was staying up
in Tollcross, and I got a job dishwashing. They saw my arms – the
scratches, the wounds. My boss said if I don't get a sick certificate from
the doctor, he won't give me a job. So I went down to the Royal Ed in a
taxi. The psychiatrist said, "You are depressed, aren't you?"

I got sectioned for one month. I had to take anti-depressants. I was
drinking wine, and I vomited in my room. I was in debt with my bank,
I was buying more wine and bringing it back onto the ward. I got
released a month later, then I got a hostel in Leith. I was still hearing
voices in my head.

I thought, nothing is going right in my life, everything's going wrong,
what have I done to deserve this? So I went back to the cult in
Edinburgh. I got in touch with the cult leader – we met at Burger King.
It had been two months since I'd left the cult in Leeds. I said, "I've got
problems," and the leader in Edinburgh said, "What do you want me to
do about it? Do you want to come back?" And I said, "yeah".

I went round to his house, he cooked a meal. I was the only Black person there. I got racially provoked there – somebody said, "I feel sorry for you Black people." And the leader didn't do nothing about it. The leader was my mentor. He gave me tasks to do – get jobs, go on courses – and he still wouldn't let me in.

I was living in a homeless hostel. I got picked on there. They call me names; when the phone rings – my mum ringing me – people aren't knocking on my door saying there's a phone call for you, people are just hanging up the phone.

Two months later I got reinstated to the cult. I was still hearing voices.

I had a social worker at the time, because of all the problems I was having with the cult. She got me a flat and a grant to buy furniture.

The leader tried to pressure me to go into a brothers' flat. I said I'd get abused again, like I did in Leeds and London. He said I'd get peace, security, the brothers will pay your rent. I said no, I don't think so, because the brothers in Leeds owe me over six grand, in rent arrears and bounced cheques. So he said, "You might as well leave." I said, "I'm not leaving, I'm alright".

I know somebody that committed suicide in London, in the cult. I nearly died myself once. I took an overdose of anti-depressants – I was found unconscious in my bed, and the cult took me to hospital in the ambulance. When I came around, the ward round doctors were in my room; they said I'm lucky to be alive, if I'd taken more anti-depressants I would be dead.

Just before I left the cult, the leader said, "I'll clean your evil spirit". At a meeting he said, "You're sick". So I decided to leave. I said my goodbyes for the last time. I went home, and that was it, I left them for good.

Wow, that must have taken a lot of strength.
Aye. My social worker said, "These are bullies. I'll get you in touch with the Cult Helpline, you can meet up at the Royal Edinburgh Hospital." After I left, the cult kept ringing me five times a day for six weeks, they kept coming round to my flat, putting notes through my front door saying, "We care about you, come back." So when I got in touch with the Cult Helpline, they wrote the cult a letter saying, "If you don't back off we'll take you to court." And they finally left me alone.

I moved houses, had nine failed tenancies, I got in trouble with the police. Three neighbours from hell called me "black bastard", so I got a bottle and hit one of them over the head with it, and I got arrested for that.

Police said he'd smash my face in if I tried anything. He put my face up against the wall and put the cuffs on me, and I got frog-marched down to the police station and put in the cell. They took my glasses off me.

I got evicted from my flat. I was put in a high rise flat half a mile down the road from the incident. I bumped into him in the post office – the victim that I hit with the bottle. He said someone's going to kill me. I went and slashed my wrists. I was hearing voices; I was really frightened. The police came round, and took me to hospital to get stitches.

I had a lawyer, and I had a witness who came to my defence at the trial. I spent two nights in Saughton Prison during my three day GBH trial. They said, "We find you guilty of assault under provocation." The verdict was unanimous. I got a year's probation.

I got involved in drugs. I became a drug dealer, I was smoking weed, hash, heroin, cocaine. I was in the Royal Ed in 1999, just before my trial.

How long were you there for that time?
Two months. I spent the Millennium in the hospital. I got a girlfriend, I got engaged, she pawned the engagement ring for a bottle of vodka, we split up.

I moved into supported accommodation. I had to give up my cats – I was crying when I gave them up. I got abused by staff – they shouted at me. I was racially provoked by one of the visitors, who called me 'n*gger' and 'black bastard'.

After a couple more moves I moved into another supported accommodation. They said they'll pay my debts off for me. For six weeks I had no money to live off, and after that I had to clean my room before I got my five pounds. I was shouting and swearing at them, and they gave me a hard time. I was in and out of the Royal Ed. I was hearing voices saying to kill one of the workers who was really horrible to me.

My mum passed away, in 2008. I went down to London. I got pickpocketed by two sex workers. My family treated me bad. They cut me out – I wasn't put in the funeral programme. My uncle said if I touch any of my mum's heritage he'd break both my legs.

After we buried my mum I came back to Edinburgh. I got a flat at the Grassmarket. I got a horrible CPN. He dumped me in hospital for two weeks, no reason. I was smoking cocaine in the toilets. Then they said to me they're going to take my money off me, give me a budget. So I said them on the answering machine, "If you attempt to take my money I'll kill the lot of you". So they came round with the police, at my front door – my CPN was there, my social worker was there, my shrink was there. I got arrested and got put in Meadows Ward for ten months. Then the rehab ward, Craiglea, for four years. So I was left sharing a room with people, who would take my stuff.

Was there anything in the hospital that helped you to feel well, or get well?
I was even worse.

You felt worse in there?
They put me on depot injections, and took me off it. They put me on tablets, and it didn't work. They put me on Compazine, that didn't work, then they put me on what I'm taking now. I get it once a week.

And does it help you now?
A little bit. I kept on running away to Dundee, with my bus pass, kept staying in hospital overnight, at Ninewells. The staff from Craiglea had to come and pick me up and take me back to the ward.

Why did you go to Ninewells? Was it better?
A lot better. You got your own room, your own shower, your own toilet. Food's a lot better. Patients are a lot better up there. There's no racism, they'll look after your cigarettes. They look out for each other up there.

In Craiglea, I was carrying diabetes and it was never detected. They didn't detect it until I was here in supported accommodation and I started going blind. I had three insulin shock fits.

So you left Craiglea and came here – how did you get discharged?
I was complying with my injections, I felt better. I was ready to move.

And then what was it like to move here?
A bit strange – really hard. I was away for four years. I was sharing a flat upstairs with a flatmate. I felt a bit lonely so I moved downstairs. But staff being in my room, I don't like it. I want to move. I want control of my money, my bus pass, my cigarettes. It's a bit like hospital really.

And is there anything that helps you to be well here?
Just the injection.

Was there a turning point, somebody that helped you, or a moment that helped?
The Cult Helpline helped me. When I first got admitted to the Royal Ed, I had a social worker and that was it – not a lot of support. I still had feelings for the cult I was in, so I went back to the cult as soon as I got discharged from the Royal Ed. When I finally left them and wanted to leave for good, my social worker put me in touch with the Cult Helpline. They supported me for three years.

What advice would you give to people running a hospital, or a place like your supported accommodation?
People can control their money, stick to their budget, have their bank cards. My money's being controlled. If they give me my bank card I'd stick to my budget every week, bring back receipts.

What would you say your hopes and dreams are? What do you hope for the future?
I'd like to write scripts for films.

And what do you think is the most important lesson life has taught you?
I've come out stronger. I've been through a lot. All the abuse I've been
through has made me stronger. Even though I get times when I get low,
and hurt myself.

*So things are still difficult sometimes. When you're feeling bad, is there
anything that helps?*
I go on YouTube, listen to loud music, heavy metal. Maybe go on
holiday somewhere, or maybe go on a day trip somewhere, like North
Berwick.

*What advice would you give to someone who was being admitted to hospital
now?*
Be positive you will get out. Comply with your medication. Don't
drink alcohol on the ward. Get a social worker, try and get placed
somewhere, get supported accommodation or a flat. Don't take drugs.

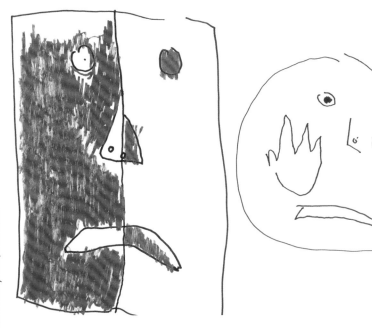

Bou Bou Synnar, *Beelzebub*

I'm flying like an eagle

Bou Bou Synnar

I'm flying
I'm flying
I'm flying like an eagle
The fish in the sea
Pacific ocean
I'm flying
I'm flying
I'm flying like an eagle
I'm swimming with dolphins
Chasing sharks in the sea
I'm flying
I'm flying
I'm flying like an eagle
The birds in the sky
They fly real high
I'm flying
I'm flying
I'm flying like an eagle
The flowers blossoming
They blossom in the spring

A NON

The Story of my Life

I was literally saved and reborn thanks to the NHS and the Royal Edinburgh Hospital. I had taken care of my parents for a very long time; unfortunately their health had deteriorated to such an extent that they had to live in an old age nursing home.

My parents have passed away now. They were born in Madagascar, under the French colonial rule, in the 1930s. My father was a physician, a GP; he had had to leave Madagascar to study medicine in Paris. His father, my grandfather, was also a physician and a GP. Both my parents were born and spent their childhood in the capital of Madagascar, Antananarivo; Antananarivo is on the highlands of Madagascar, with an altitude of about 900 metres.

My mother was also born in Antananarivo; she was a really artistic lady. She was a passionate pianist: she also left Madagascar to study the piano. She was also gifted in foreign languages; she taught me English when I was seven. She had to do all sorts of jobs to finance her musical studies. She graduated as an English and French secretary; she was a student of piano at the Ecole Normale de Musique, in Paris, under the guidance of Alfred Cortot and Robert Manuel.

I would not say that I had a happy childhood. Since Kindergarten I had to deal with rejection, ostracism, racism. I was always one of the top pupils and top students; being good at my studying was one way to assert myself. I had poor self-esteem, I was constantly bullied and mocked by the other pupils.

Things changed radically after my first stay in England. My brother and I spent three weeks in England, in Wittering, as boarding guests. My very first childhood love was American, she was blonde and blue-eyed.

So, my brother and I were on

our own, strolling in London. I was twelve and my brother was nine. We were in Carnaby Street, Picadilly Circus, Buckingham Palace.

London in 1972 was a fascinating place. The Beatles were still singing together, mini skirts were in fashion, the Austin Cooper Mini cars were also hitting the roads.

I got good grades in English, as we were given English courses. I also did some boat sailing, one or two years later, in Southampton.

Every year, my parents, my brother and I spent our summer holidays in Spain.

What can I remember from the 1970s? The smell of car petrol, on the highways, the feeling that everything was possible. We had black and white TV sets, the American Vietnam War was going full blast, we saw the 1968 student demonstrations in Paris, the Black Panthers in the USA, the first landing on the moon in July 1969.

Spain was still under the iron rule of General Franco. As tourist kids we did not understand much about it. I was soon able to speak Spanish. We had holidays in Alicante, Almeria, Tenerife, Majorca.

I had my first mental health problems in 1978. I just had some kind of nervous breakdown, mental depression.

Years later, a girl who was in my junior high school told me that some pupils had put some drugs in my drinks during the lunch at the dining room.

1978 was the year of my French A levels, my Baccalaureat. I had to sit the September examination.

Later on, I did my French military service during one whole year, at the Ecole Militaire in Paris, serving as a translator, interpreter, and instructor for English. I worked with the American military attaché and the British military attaché.

Some of the French officers did not like me. They bullied me and I ended up in a French Military Hospital, in Percy, in the suburbs of Paris.

My mother visited me every day. I was sharing a room with two other guys from Madagascar. My Mum brought us some nice Madagascan meals.

Our home was in Orly ville, near the Orly Airport. I have vivid memories of waiting for our Grandmother, who was flying from Madagascar with the Boeing 707 of Air Madagascar. In those days we could watch and literally experience the landings of all the aircraft.

My life was going on; I graduated from the Paris University, the Sorbonne, I did a Masters Degree in North American, British and Irish studies, specialising in Asian Americans and Chinese Americans. I also did an MBA at Regents College in Regents Street in London.

I spent about eleven years of my life in Germany, in Hamburg, Ingolstadt and Duesseldorf, as I had also graduated from the European Business School in Reichartshausen, in Oestrich Winkel, near Frankfurt on the Main.

I realise now that all my health problems are really some blessings in disguise. Like the German philosopher Nietzsche wrote, all things which do not kill you make you stronger.

One of my great uncles from Madagascar studied medicine at the Royal Edinburgh Hospital. I had to stay at the Orchard Clinic, Cedar Ward, but my old aunties had told me so much about the Royal Ed and Florence Nightingale, that I already knew the place. Thanks to the wonderful work of the OTs and the doctors I realized there was a pattern in my mental health problems.

Resilience, empathy, understanding other people's cultures and way of life; all these things are a part of me now.

The wonderful people from free advocacy were also instrumental in my recovering.

I have given up hatred towards anybody. Every day is a new day, a new life. I am going to apply for British citizenship.

I would like to say, like Prince Harry did, that there is no shame in asking for professional help for mental problems. The stigma attached to mental health issues has to be destroyed. Seeking professional help is always the best solution.

But there is a spiritual dimension linked to these issues. Once we see the greater picture, once we understand the real meanings of our sufferings, we are free.

As it is said in the Bible "and the truth shall set you free".

Medications, psychotherapy, counselling, coaching are all good. But, indeed, we are our best medicine, we are our best doctors.

Once we realize that there is a supreme power, that nothing ever happens in vain, we are getting better and better. Our body might be frail, but our mind is always strong.

Upheavals, crises, sufferings, problems of all kinds should be welcomed with open arms. We are Vikings of life, the hard wind from the North makes us ever stronger, there is no limit to what we can do.

Let us have faith in God, let us have faith in humanity, let us choose life.

Day by day, step by step, drop by drop, we are on our journey in life.

Yesterday is gone, tomorrow is a dream, all we have is the present. The present is the best present. We should fear no loss, we shall expect no reward, freedom is in accepting all that may occur.

As a final word, I would like to state that there is a life after this life. I was declared clinically dead twice, and both times I met my grandmother who told me I had to go back to this world.

To the young people, as one who has suffered much and seen much, I want to stress that smoking, all kinds of smoking, alcohol and all intoxicating substances should be avoided.

So, God bless you all, and let us keep going, enjoying the journey of life,

Yours, go brae,

A NON

ALBERT STEWART NICOLSON

Taking a Trip Down Memory Lane

Walking with angels, I filled in for fools
My conflict of interest broke all the rules
Being thrice blessed is quite an adventure
The problem inherent in decades of censure
Not being just human became quite a drag
Transcendence in Being was my trusty bag
A lifetime surviving, what did I know
Brain jacketed straight, how did I grow
The psyche is mind soul and spirit
Living with nature over their limit
Matter as content a mirror in nature
Heredity surely as instinct a feature
Beyond their preserve is just not allowed
Truth would all out, of an unholy shroud
Doors open can welcome cathartic relief
Centuries of wisdom enhanced by belief
Holding a candle through infinite night
Opens a path through treasured insight

JO McFARLANE INTERVIEWS MERRICK POPE

Drawing strength from one another

I first met Merrick (but didn't set eyes on her till a year later) in 2004 when she worked on the Psychiatric Emergency Team (PET) based at the Royal Edinburgh Hospital. My social worker Heather Millar had visited me one evening when I was in crisis and felt that I should be admitted to hospital, so she 'persuaded' me to come with her to be assessed by PET.

I was very reluctant to do so as I had had some unpleasant experiences of the mental health assessment service in the past which caused me to feel even worse after I called them. Being reprimanded and made to feel like a time-waster exacerbated my paranoia, shame and despair and it precipitated future suicide attempts because I felt there was nowhere safe to turn.

Statutory services seem to operate on the assumption that if you ask for help you mustn't need it; and if you refuse their 'help' when it's imposed, you must be psychotic and need to be sectioned. It's a cruel paradox whichever side of the equation you are on. I was in no hurry to test out my status as either 'deluded' or 'malingerer'. I hate being in hospital but was frightened of being left to the mercy of my self-destructive impulses at home so neither outcome was desirable (this was in the days before intensive home treatment teams (IHTTs)).

Heather assured me that I would be taken seriously and given the help I needed - not necessarily hospital, and if so, only for a short admission this time. She had promised this before and was left with egg on her face when they subjected me to a stern, humiliating cross examination even with her present, then were happy to let me run off into the nearest car because I was so frightened. Heather, of course, was horrified and angry but powerless to influence them even though she had known me for 10 years and they didn't know me at all. Needless to say I ended up in hospital in Oxford the next day following a near fatal overdose.

So it was a huge risk for us both to put ourselves (Heather's professional judgement and my life) at their mercy. But Heather insisted so I had to be practically frog-marched down to the hospital. Fortunately, Merrick was the nurse on duty that night and she treated me with great tenderness and care, helping to restore my trust in the system.

In typical humility and openness, Merrick has now offered to be 'assessed' by me for this book.

Jo: I met you back in 2004, when you worked on the Psychiatric Emergency Team. What caused you to admit me that night?

Merrick: What I remember was that it was a decision that I took really very quickly; that there didn't need to be a whole load of explanation as to the distress that you were in, it was quite evident. And my concern for you at that time, given the experiences that you'd had in the past, was that you were really at high risk of killing yourself. Hospital was the best place for you, as hard and as horrible as hospital can sometimes be. I don't know what you remember about that night?

Jo: There was a pull-push thing going on for me, because I hate being in hospital, and I've had some bad experiences, but at the same time, there's that terror of feeling so suicidal – I wanted to jump out of the window, which is a real risk for me, because I jumped off Salisbury Crags. And so I just felt in a great deal of danger. So although I didn't want to be in hospital, and couldn't make that decision myself, I needed yourself and Heather to make that decision for me and keep me safe.

Merrick: I think you're right – there's that difficulty of somebody's rights and wishes, versus – sometimes I think we all just want someone to tell us what to do, and make that decision for us. And it's not that that's ideal all the time in life, but every now and again I think it's OK.

Jo: The problem is when people get kept in a 'sick' role for long periods of time. But sometimes if that intervention is made in a crisis, it can help you then to take that responsibility for your own life. I was wondering how it feels for you, or how it felt at that time, to have that kind of power over someone's fate, knowing what the risks are?

Merrick: Within the emergency team, you're right, it is a power, and it's something that you have to respect. It's not just about you coming into hospital; that then takes away your ability to choose what time you see people, what time you have visitors, when you can go for a bath – the power extends and ripples out. Some things you have to do in an emergency, you had very little time to think about it, but you have to sit with the consequences of it.

Jo: I don't know if you've ever experienced someone being turned away, and losing them to suicide and how that felt or would feel? I know that's a difficult question.

Merrick: When I worked in PET it was actually easier if you admitted somebody. That sits easier because you're actually doing something – it was harder to say that this isn't the right place for you. But thankfully when I worked in PET, there was nobody I assessed who then went out and killed themselves. Which I was very lucky about, I think – whether that's because I was more cautious, or it was just that it never happened when I worked. But I've worked with people who went on to complete suicide: either I've been directly involved in their care, or in the peripheries of their care – and it's devastating.

I do an MBT [mentalisation-based treatment] therapy group and somebody was really surprised that we feel for our patients. They said actually, we thought this was just a job to you.

Jo: And it's quite clear to me that you do really care, and you've a lot invested emotionally in the people you work with.

Merrick: I think the people who come across as if they don't care – it's about being curious as to why that is. Is it a defence mechanism for them? I don't think people really come into this job to brutalise people. Realistically, what's happened to them in the process of their career that's resulted in them turning into Nurse Ratchett?

Jo: In terms of assessing people on that team, I think often when you decide not to make an intervention, just listening and being kind to someone in the way you deal with them can help that person go away feeling OK about themselves – and they maybe didn't necessarily need anything to happen but that.

Sometimes as a patient it can feel quite arbitrary, being on the receiving end of that decision. I was wondering what are the criteria for being admitted to hospital, or being referred to IHTT?

Merrick: I haven't worked in the assessment service since 2005, so a lot has changed since then. There are a lot less beds. So the folk who are coming into hospital now – you have to be really acutely unwell. And any sense of sanctuary, or respite, isn't really there within an acute admission ward any longer. So there isn't as far as I'm aware any written criteria; it's more about where there's risk to yourself, risk to other people, whether you're neglecting to look after yourself, whether there's medication that doesn't seem to be working.

Jo: So a really difficult time to do the job. How much do you think people assessing would be influenced by the person's diagnosis, by their reputation in services? Or even whether the person likes you or dislikes you when they meet you?

Merrick: I think the party line would be that somebody's diagnosis, reputation, likeability, should have nothing to do with it. However, some of the women I work with, they tell me they have sense that their reputation goes before them, or they're viewed through the prism of their diagnosis.

There's no other client group that would get spoken about, or denied or accepted for treatment, in the same way that folk who are given the kind of diagnosis that folk that I work with get – which is Borderline Personality Disorder (BPD) or Emotionally Unstable Personality Disorder (EUPD). But it's still part of the culture in some places that it's OK to be derogatory about folk who have been given this diagnosis. And how does that happen?

Jo: That begs me to wonder as we look forward, is the diagnostic model helpful? Or should we be ditching that and thinking about people's distress in a different way, and how we treat it and understand it?

Merrick: Certainly for BPD, there's 256 variables for what that might be, because you have to tick positive for five out of nine criteria, so you can have five and I can have five, and we've only got one overlapping. And so we could have entirely different experiences. So it's more about what's happening for you, rather than what's your label, I would say. And likewise two people can have entirely difference experiences of psychosis or a mood disorder.

Jo: Your role now is to support people who self-harm. What motivates you in that role?

Merrick: The people that I work with, most definitely. When I did my training, we got two hours around self-harm in a three-year training. And nothing around personality development, let alone personality disorder.

I started working in the acute admissions ward as my first post. I could feel myself turning into somebody that I didn't like – because I'm trying to fit in, it's my first job in the Royal Ed and people were saying to me "you're getting sucked in by them" and "they're manipulating you" – whereas I really actually enjoyed working with women who had that kind of presentation – and so I had that moment of clarity – of wow, stop the bus.

In 2005, I was asked if I would do a three-month secondment to think about what could be improved around working with folk who self-harm. That secondment was extended and extended – so here we are now, in 2017. What I did in the first days was a scoping exercise, with people who use services and with staff and with carers, to try and build a service that people actually wanted, rather than imposing something on people.

It's quite dynamic in what's being offered. There are things that are set in stone, like facilitated peer support groups, and everything else kind of gets built around them. I do individual clinic work with folk who are inpatients, and sometimes I will see folk individually for a short period of time in transitioning back home as well – because being in hospital can be hard, but going back home can be hard too. I do a variety of outpatient bits and bobs: support groups, a creative writing group. Every year I have a research project as well, and I do quite a lot of teaching.

Jo: They certainly get their money's worth out of you! Your passion for it shines through, really. What aspects do you find most challenging about your job?

Merrick: I think the fact that it's me, working thirty hours a week, on a budget of zero pence, can sometimes be a bit of a challenge, because the remit of the role is so huge.

What I realised is what a massive ancient juggernaut the NHS is. It's generational change really. I came into the job with, as I described it, my Baader-Meinhof mentality of kicking the tables. But I realised too that I could be outside the NHS chucking stones at it or I could be inside it, changing it person by person.

Jo: Have there been changes that you have noticed in how people who self-harm are treated and understood, since you've started?

Merrick: I think so. I think there is more of an awareness and an understanding that this is coming from somewhere – that somebody is not self-harming at eight o'clock at night to annoy you, that that's been driven by distress.

There's been a change in the generation of nurses since the Mental Health Act changed in the 2000s and folk who were given a personality disorder diagnosis were encompassed in the Act. I think some of the doctors are becoming more psychologically-minded, rather than just the medical model as well. Whether that actually translates into what folk who use services might say, is a different thing.

Jo: You have very good relationships with people you work with – I can say that as someone who you've worked with. People trust you and feel really listened to and understood. What do you think makes a difference?

Merrick: I view it as – we're two people, sitting in a room together. It's not about me telling somebody what to do. I don't live through my job title, if that makes sense. "There but for the grace of God go

I"; it might be me, in the other chair. I'm aware of how fragile good mental health can be. I hope to be a human being with somebody, rather than a nurse bot.

Jo: That's so evident in you: you really treat people as equals and with great humanity. How do you manage when it's all getting on top of you?

Merrick: I have supervision once a week, and I appreciate that is it incredibly rare for nurses to have an hour out every single week. So I have lots of opportunity to think about my thinking. I have a world outside the hospital as well, and I can transition quickly into that – there are other people that need me outside of hospital, and that focuses you. I've done a lot of mindfulness practice as well, so I incorporate bits and bobs like that. Playing *Candy Crush* helps to switch off too…

Jo: Thank goodness for *Candy Crush*, if it helps you to do your job! The last thing we want is for people to get burnt out and overwhelmed by the demands of the role.

What still needs to change, in terms of how people who self-harm or have that diagnosis of BPD are treated in the system?

Merrick: I think it comes back to education. Self-harm is just a symptom. How people are trying to cope should be considered – I think that there need to be, ideally, more sophisticated responses, if we do want to use a diagnostic model. Whether an acute admission ward is the best place for that to happen, is a whole other conversation as well – or whether it's somewhere that works in a more therapeutic, community, psychologically minded way.

Jo: I agree with that. Why do you think there has been such stigma and misunderstanding around people that you work with?

Merrick: I think most of us do fairly negative stuff to try and up our mood state. We eat too much, we drink, we smoke fags, we pick a fight with our partner that's actually about something else. I think it's really interesting how society has homed in on the folk who do the visible things like cut and burn themselves and get their knickers in a twist about that, as opposed to all the other stuff that everybody else is doing but aren't stigmatized for.

Jo: Do you think there is a bit of scapegoating that goes on?

Merrick: Yes. I think sometimes the things that folk do if they have difficulties with impulsivity and anger, I think there is something that touches us on a deeper level. I don't think there is anybody that hasn't got a parking ticket and doesn't want to go straight into the City Chambers and slap it down and tell them to eff off! We close that down and go "that's terrible," but actually there is a little bit in us that goes, "I wish I could do that." I think cultures who are more openly expressive – that's maybe a good thing. Rather than our repressed Scottish mentality.

Jo: For me, there is something very liberating about having a mad identity. I feel that in some ways it's been a bit of a passport to be able to be more authentic and actually explore what it is that I want, and not having to fit in. So I think there is a freedom in madness.

Merrick: You know, I maybe mirror that in part – in that I'm not entirely sure the hospital knew what do with me: who I am and how I work and how I think. I think that I was very lucky to be given the freedom to develop this role. I'm not very good at taking orders; I think I would struggle to work in a hierarchy of a ward. So allowing me to be me in my work, has allowed this service to develop in part as well.

Jo: I think there is a price to pay for not falling in line with the culture. I remember being on the ward years ago, there was a lovely, lovely nurse. She really spoke to the patients and was very gentle and kind, and I actually saw her being really ostracised by the other nurses on the ward – they were making bitchy comments about her, which we weren't supposed to hear. It made me think that actually it's very hard, as a professional working in a system like that, in a culture like that, to be able to keep up your own humanity and not to fall in with the negative aspects of that culture.

I'm trying to empathize with that – what's it like to be a nurse in that situation. I was in a hospital for four years when I was younger, and there were quite a lot of bad things happened. I was a very angry young woman and I had a real sense of, this is really unjust, and I spoke out against it. I didn't always deal with it in the best way; I got angry and lashed out. Then I noticed that when I was in hospital a couple of years later, that edge to me went. Part of it is growing older – a lot of the angry young woman thing goes. But I'm ashamed to say I didn't stand up for people. I had to do that in order to survive, to get some sort of care in there. I've always felt really bad about that. So I can understand, in a way, what it must be like for staff working in that situation: to become co-opted into that culture, and for it to be too much of a heavy price to stand up for what you believe in.

Merrick: Doing surveys with folk when I started out, what the staff were saying mirrored what the folk who were in wards and using the services were saying. About what they wanted from the services, how they wanted the services to be developed, what their failings were.

Jo: Looking at the history of psychiatry and mental health services, there have been fundamental paradigm shifts. From moral treatment and people who worked in hospitals being called attendants and then suddenly, last century, being medicalised and then becoming nurses. Is it possible to have another major paradigm shift? Is it more nurses and psychiatrists we need? Or is it something different?

Merrick: Mental health nurses have to have a think about what their role is. Our job has changed. Previously we were involved in lots of different types of therapies and now, psychology has a much bigger presence in the hospital settings. OTs [Occupational Therapists] do lots of the roles that nurses used to do. So who are the nurses now? It's difficult when there are very few nurses on, and there is a locked door, and everybody wants out for fags. They are policing the wards, looking for people smoking, rather than using some of the skills that they have been trained in. I think we need to have a think about, what are we needed for? Because it would be horrific if we went back to being attendants and just having a custodial function on somebody's liberty.

Jo: What idea or book or person has most inspired you?

Merrick: Man's Search for Meaning by Viktor Frankl. It's a really short book, but he was the founding father of existential psychotherapy and he says, "If man has a why to live, he can survive the how." When you are questioning that, either in your own life or your professional life, it's a really useful book to just go back to. I think we all need to have a sense of purpose in life, and a sense of responsibility, and of being needed and loved and cared for. I would say that that has been quite influential in my thinking, both within work and out.

Jo: I love *Man's Search for Meaning* as well – it's one of my favourite books, it's very beautiful. And what book or person do you find most difficult or challenging or repellent?

Merrick: Somebody who I was repelled by as an angry young woman, which has informed some of my thinking and who I am today, is Maggie Thatcher. I'm a child of the Thatcher era. I met my best friend on the first day of university, when we were going to share a room together – she had come down from Lewis and arrived to find me hammering a 'Pay No Poll Tax' poster on to our communal door, with no discussion or negotiation.

Jo: Did she agree with you?

Merrick: I think she was a bit startled! It was how the Thatcher era viewed societies and communities and destroyed aspects of those – that sense of "You have to sort this out for yourself." And, as far as I could tell, an utter lack of compassion. I think it spurred me on into being quite political when I was younger, and I think the job that I do now in some ways is a political job, in that I champion and fight for the person at the bottom of the heap. I think that psychiatry does have a kind of hierarchy of diagnoses and the people that I work with seem to be fairly near the bottom of that, and in people's thinking or compassion or care.

Jo: Reflected in the fact that there is only one of you, doing a massive job. Are there any last words you have for people reading this?

Merrick: I would say, read the book with an open mind. Be curious about it. Be curious about where people's thinking comes from. If you are somebody who is delivering services, accept what people are saying. Don't get defensive if there are criticisms or observations: those are valid, even if you don't agree with them. It's wondering why that person is reflecting in that way on what you are trying to do or what you are trying to deliver. Talk to people.

Jo: I find you really inspirational, Merrick. Having this conversation just enhances that, not that it needed enhancing!

Merrick: Well, I think we are very lucky because we've worked together always as equals.

Jo: Definitely. I've always felt that.

Merrick: In the time that I admitted you, but also the things that we have done together.

Jo: You were able to see past that. When we first met, I didn't know what you looked like for a year because I couldn't look up at people, I was too frightened of the thoughts that were going on. You came up to me in the corridor and said "Oh, hi Jo" – you might not have been aware that I didn't know what you looked like – and that really touched me. Ever since then, you've never seen me as that broken person, but at the same time, you've always treated me with sensitivity and the care of knowing that there is that vulnerability there – but it's not all that you see.

Merrick: No, it doesn't define you.

If there is a downfall of admitting somebody, it can be that the mental health services are Kafkaesque: really difficult to get into and then impossible to get out of. I'm glad that you have a world and a life that has nothing to do with the Royal Ed. You are an artist and a poet and a writer and everything else.

Jo: And I've discharged myself from psychiatry, which feels brilliant. Nearly 28 years, and I'm free of psychiatry – and it feels great. I've got something for you. I've got something to present Merrick with, on tape. I think it's appropriate.

[Jo gives Merrick a Wonder Woman mug and pants set]

Merrick: I hope they are a large size!

Jo: It just seems very apt for you.

Merrick: Well thank you very much for that, Jo.

Jo: Doing all that in thirty hours a week, I don't know how you do it, it's amazing.

Merrick: You know what I think – if people were just kind to each other, not just in hospital, but everywhere, across society, we would be much better for it.

Jo: What I love about what you have been saying, is that where you see things that are challenging in terms of attitudes and practices, it's about trying to understand and not to blame – to try and understand where people are coming from.

Merrick: Yes. I think you get a better result – trying to get that person to understand what their role in that is, and that it's not too late to change for them. Sometimes they have taken on their crabbit identity.

Jo: I think it would take a lot of courage. I would imagine for a lot of people who have worked for a long time in that service, the mammoth shift in attitude and getting to grips with new understanding, plus the new things that are thrown in the system. It must take a lot of courage to change, as it would for all of us.

JO MᶜFARLANE

Illegitimi

I arrived at reception a sorry mess
No hope of my passing the gatekeeper's test
The waiting room grubby with outcasts like me
Too sick for a cure, too well to be seen

The doctor eventually called out my name
Pronouncing it wrong... relief all the same
The cliffs in my head were too scary to mention
She seemed nonetheless to pick up my intention

"Suicide isn't a mental illness
You're not a priority, none of our business
The voluntary sector's where you should go
They've got plenty of time for a waster like you"

JO McFARLANE

A Good Experience of Being Sectioned

"Well here you are now
and you're in the right place
Though I don't have your notes
and I'm new to your case
It's clear to the eye
you are very distressed
You need some attention,
a safe place to rest

I'm going to admit you
for a minimum spell
Till you're back on your feet
and you start to feel well
With a bed for the night
and people who care
Tomorrow won't seem
such a hellish nightmare"

Dedicated to Merrick Pope

White Coats

They read my psychosis as though it were a sonnet
or the prelude to some operatic outburst.
They tell me Take the tablets! and I do.
We all agree they make me better.
They slay my insane thoughts like doves on an altar.
Voices of unreason scavenge the remains.

The white coats without white coats
confer behind glass doors,
decide if I am well enough to leave the ward.
They form a scrum so mysterious and compelling
that I watch and listen for their every move;
circumnavigate the outcome, play my part.

Psychiatrists are wise as trees, upright as a Sunday stroll
along the promenade; seldom careless as a door unlatched,
seldom unassuming. Never wrong. They are coming to free me
from my prison; SHOCK ME with their peculiar brand of truth.
It goes like this: I am a patient in a psychiatric hospital
and they are here to help me.

Then where are the white coats, the couch,
and the pendulum? Where is the dictum
of reason that holds me here, will later let me go?
Is it written in their superlative smiles,
their shiny suits,
their conveyer belt of consultations?

They tell me to trust them, and I do.

JODI

We believe recovery is possible for everyone

I am a Peer Worker for mental health charity Penumbra. I am based within the rehabilitation ward Myreside in the Royal Edinburgh Hospital and also work at Firrhill, which is a community based residence for people who have recently been discharged from hospital.

Firrhill and Myreside are both part of a project called Progressing on Both Fronts (PoBF). It is a partnership involving Penumbra, who offer peer support; Carr Gomm, who offer living support services; Edinburgh Volunteer Centre; and the NHS. We work as part of a large multi-disciplinary team aiming to help individuals to develop skills, confidence and resilience so they can move back into the community.

As a Peer Worker, I have experienced my own struggle with mental ill health in the past. I now use this as part of my job, and my own experience of recovery is considered an asset when offering support to people. The relationships I have with each individual are based on mutuality and personal understanding. I promote recovery and use a strengths-based approach which focuses on personal qualities, abilities, interests and beliefs. I help people to identify goals and milestones which are important to them - the question I ask most is 'What is important to you?'

Every individual is different, but one of Penumbra's core beliefs is that recovery is possible for everyone. There are individuals who are very unwell and experience symptoms which cause them distress on a daily basis, but we hope all individuals are gradually making progress in managing their symptoms and lives.

The most important part of my job as a Peer Worker in Firrhill and Myreside is the relationship I have with each person.

Relationships last for quite a long time (2 years+) and you need consistency and perseverance. I offer a lot of encouragement to people, helping them to stay motivated in their interests and activities. This involves reinforcing their strengths and talents (many people are extremely creative and talented!), offering emotional support, and challenging barriers and obstacles.

I think it is important to recognise each person as an individual (not a diagnosis!), and to offer hope that recovery is possible, no matter how small the steps or changes are.

Being a Peer Worker in Firrhill and Myreside is certainly not without its challenges! I aim to get as many people as possible involved in activities in the community, although this is not always easy. Some people have been in hospital for a long time and are fearful to leave the ward. Progress can be slow, although when we finally do manage to overcome a barrier or obstacle it is a real success. That is the thing about recovery that I always aim to promote within my peer relationships, that no matter how small the goal you want to achieve, once you finally achieve it you will feel on top of the world! We always like to celebrate progress.

My role within Firrhill and Myreside is also about promoting independence, encouraging self care, and getting people to believe in their own potential! We use the Penumbra I•ROC tool (Individual Recovery Outcomes Measure) within both services to help people identify areas of life they would like to improve. This can include social network, personal strengths, qualities and values, family links, self management, hopes for the future, and much more. I•ROC also helps us to evaluate the progress people are making with their recovery.

As a Peer Worker, the mutuality within the peer relationship allows for a great deal of honesty and authenticity, both from them and me. The people I support know I have been there, and have had similar experiences to them – from living with symptoms to hospital admissions. People are always asking questions about my own experience of mental ill health. Many have said that it was really helpful for them to hear about a personal experience – they can really identify with it, and it encourages the belief that recovery is possible for everyone. For me, that is what makes the peer relationship unique and special – we can learn from each other.

Peer work is so rewarding because it allows us to walk alongside people in both the good and bad times, it allows us to hold the hope for individuals when they are struggling, and to be there beside them when they overcome challenging times.

I help by sharing self management techniques and recovery tips and ideas, offering suggestions and emotional support while reminding individuals of their strengths, progress and resilience to cope in times of adversity. We look together at what works to keep individuals well, and what support individuals may require to help improve their mental health and wellbeing.

Peer work is a really enjoyable job and the best part about it is seeing how truly compassionate and courageous people are. The people I support never fail to ask me how I am doing or how my week has been, and they are always quick to reach out to others in need - their compassion knows no end.

I have found that showing compassion and listening is one of the most important parts of being a Peer Worker. People have shared with me how distressing it can be when they are experiencing voices or side-effects from medication. Sometimes the best thing I can do is to just listen and be there to walk alongside them when they experience difficult times - the experience of just being heard by another human being can be profoundly powerful. Sometimes I can identify with their distress from my own lived experience, sometimes I cannot – but I am always prepared to listen empathetically and remind them they are not alone.

I meet with each individual once a week to do a planned activity, either out in the community or somewhere within the hospital grounds. Activities vary from person to person, depending on their interests and goals. Some people like to play badminton, attend the gym, take occasional trips to the cinema, or sometimes just go for a nice walk in the community. Others enjoy attending music groups with me, visiting the library, gardening or simply visiting a coffee shop somewhere in the community. When people do not feel like leaving the ward, we create art work, play board games, or simply just sit and have a conversation over a cup of tea.

Penumbra promotes personal choice, and although we encourage people to participate in activities and stick to their commitments, we understand flexibility and allowing people the right to change their mind (the same way we all do) is important.

I never force anyone to do something they do not want to do. Instead we explore whether there are any barriers or challenges I can help them to overcome. This has proven to be the most effective approach.

One woman I support, for example, was reluctant to try new activities because she was scared to use public transport on her own. We practiced on the bus together at first, finding a seat where she felt most comfortable (with me sitting a few seats away from her!) and exiting the bus together. After a few goes, I asked her "How did that feel?" and she said: "I felt really nervous at first sitting there on my own, but after a while I forgot you were even there!" Now she is able to board the bus by herself and make long trips across town to visit her relatives without any support – she just makes sure she sits in her favourite seat beside the driver. She has overcome her fear of travelling alone, which has allowed her to get back into the community and build her social network. A relatively small thing (for most people) has been a big part of her recovery.

As a Peer Worker I really appreciate that even when changes or outcomes are small, they are still important steps towards building a strong foundation for recovery.

MARIANNE MᴬᶜKINTOSH

Near and Far

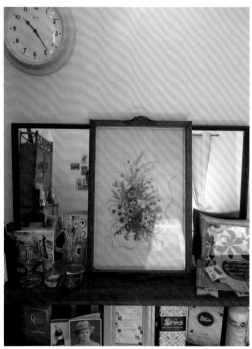
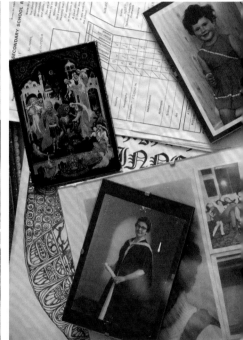

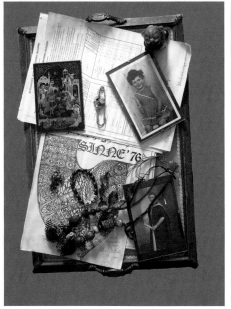
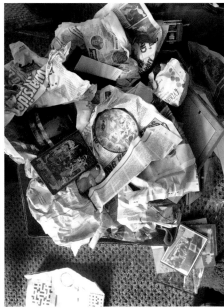
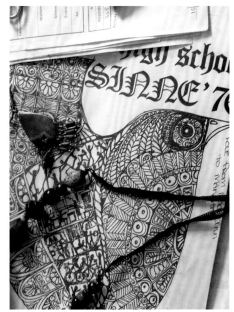

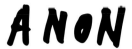

ANON

Never give up

What's your history with the hospital here?

I'll have been in the Orchard clinic for a year at the end of this month. It was very difficult to start with. I'd been looking forward to coming here so much because I had been in Carstairs for three and a half years, and that was my focus – to get here. It was difficult because I was a lot more restricted here to start with.

I don't receive any medication whatsoever, which is unusual, so a big part of my coping skills is to exercise, and I was able to do that a lot and regular in Carstairs. Plus, you've got grounds access there, because it's fenced in. You can go out with your mates and that's a great time to just relax a bit more.

There is so much peer support there, and that is important. I'm really fortunate with my family and my friends and my professional team – they are understanding – but nobody can fully understand what it's like to become unwell and commit a crime, and then to recover and have to deal with the consequences. That's where the peer support from your friends makes a massive difference. They understand it – that uncertainty, not knowing when you're going to get out. You have to be careful with that – not to let that play on your mind, because it makes day to day things more difficult.

There is a lot on offer here – loads of activities. It's great to build that up again – that makes a big massive difference to be able to do that. We go to the gym, go swimming, there's walking groups. I'm going to start playing football. It's great that it's all out in the community. The adjustment was a bit difficult to start with – to be out in the community and having to come back – but you get used to it. It's just about trying to keep that thought on being grateful: trying to focus on what I've got, as opposed to what I've not got, and realising that this is a matter of being patient. My doctor said that to me: "you'll never have to be this patient again, in your life."

What's made a big difference to me personally is my Christian faith. I've always got that. There's a really good chaplaincy service in the hospital here and they were great helping me with the adjustment of coming here. There's a lovely service every Wednesday in the hospital. I'm starting to go to church on Sunday in Morningside as well, and they have been really welcoming. And there is a spiritual group in the Orchard clinic.

What gives you hope?

Aye, that's a good question. My faith gives me hope. My family gives me hope. Other people give me hope and all. It is a really good bunch of guys here. Of course it's frustrating, but it is a good bunch of guys who're helpful and thoughtful towards each other, and that gives me hope. To see somebody that's not doing too great themselves, but they are still thinking about other people.

It's made a big difference to me, to have that faith and to have that reassurance. And hope: hope is such an important part of recovery. You've got to hold on to that.

There are a lot of people here to help, people that are genuinely interested. They just want to help your recovery and see you getting back into the community and getting back on with your life. Aye, it does make a big difference.

Mental illness affects different people in different ways. It doesn't respect the status in your life, whether you're rich or poor – and I do appreciate life better now. I was grateful and very fortunate that I had a really good life. I was happy, I was married, two beautiful kids, working, and my larger family were brilliant. My parents were brilliant too, and that's when things started to go wrong for me. A few bereavements. My mum passed away and it just got harder, my nephew passed away as well – at a young age, with cancer. It was difficult, and unfortunately I started using substances.

It took me to a really dark, dark place. Suicidal thoughts. Horrible.

You just never think it's going to start happening to you. You hear warnings about other people becoming mentally ill, going into hospital and I just thought that it would never happen to me.

Taking substances – it's just such a dangerous thing to do. You're playing Russian roulette with your mind, with your mental health, and if you have got mental health issues – thankfully I can look at it now and say – it's like pouring petrol on a fire. You're just making things so much worse, so much more unmanageable. A lot of people do that – they self-medicate. I had no idea about psychiatric hospitals, what the treatment was going to be like. I didn't know there was any help there.

I deeply regret what happened, but thankfully the person forgave me. And I was very unwell at the time. So I do feel fortunate to have a second chance, and I am confident about the future. I've got a beautiful family and I'm really lucky.

I have learned a lot, and the most important message that I could remind myself of, and to say to anybody else who is struggling, is to ask for help. You're not alone. Unfortunately, that's very common

– that's how you feel: that you are alone. But you're not. It's an illness. It's not a weakness. The stigma is changing from when I was younger, and I'm in mid-life now. There have been so many positive changes, and that is the main message that I would get over to anybody: that there is help available. You're not on your own. Once you start realising that and start getting involved in that, you hear other people and it makes a big difference – to hear from other people that have been through and come out the other end.

This experience has been humiliating, especially at the start. But it has taught me to be more humble; to have humility. Just to appreciate the simple things in life, to not to put pressure on myself.

But hey, we all struggle along sometimes, no matter who it is. You think people have got life all figured out and that they are doing great – maybe an aeroplane pilot – but he's got his problems like everybody else. We all have worries, we all have concerns, we all have insecurities, and I find it comforting just to realise that. We can help each other along and sometimes you just need to have a bit of a break. To realise that things are temporary – that this will pass – makes a massive difference.

It's great to see the new hospital – what a difference – and it's just that relief to know that there is help there for people, you'd be amazed once you find out. Especially to have that peer support. Somebody to listen, that makes a big difference – to be able to talk it through and get it out, instead of going round your own mind. Just to go, "Oh aye actually, it's not that bad. Aye, this is more manageable than I'm maybe painting it in my mind." Being kind to yourself. Take your time. It is easy to get into a rush sometimes.

I can certainly look back now and realise just how well I was doing, and… just being free. Waking up in your own house, making a cup of tea, down to the shops, getting bacon, some rolls and a paper. It's a wonderful gift, and it is easy to take that for granted. I took it for granted, like most of us do, but I'm determined to keep a hold of that and use that to my advantage.

In your recovery do you feel there was like a turning point, where things started to get better and if there was, what helped to make that turning point?

Aye, I've had a few moments like that. At first, I thought my life was over. It was really difficult to come to terms with what had happened, with how unwell I was. I'd never been in any other hospitals before in my life, I'd never had any serious mental illness. I'd had bouts of depression. I'd never had what happened to me, to become psychotic, delusional, hearing voices. Thankfully I recovered quickly from that but it's a difficult thing to come to terms with. To realise what you've actually done. Very painful. So aye, the first year was incredibly difficult and I'm very fortunate that some of my family stood by me. And that made a massive difference. My children have always been there and even when I have been really depressed, it's like that wee bit of light, that wee bit of sunshine comes through.

One of my fellow patients says to me "I found this very helpful" – and it's a wee book called *Our Daily Bread* and it is a daily Bible reading. I started reading that and there's a prayer in the back of it, and I just got down on my knees in my room and just gave my life to Jesus. I would have laughed at that ten years ago, myself. But I found that peace, I started reading the bible, started going to the Christian fellowship and they were talking about these promises. I thought, I want that – I want that peace. It worked for me. There wasn't any bolts of lightning or anything, but it's just that realisation that nah, I'm not on my own on this. And especially in Carstairs when you're locked up in your room for the night and you're on your own, just to be able to hold to that promise that no, I'm not alone. It gave me that assurance that I could hand anything over to God – my situation, my family, my friends – and I just took a lot of encouragement and hope from that.

And the psychology treatments that I've had, they've made a massive difference as well. I remember a psychologist saying to me, "You can only get out what you put in. This is up to you" – which felt a bit daunting to start with but I'm fortunate that I've got my family to keep that focus. And myself. I did, I gave it one hundred percent and they have made a massive difference to me.

The main one I did was mentalizing, for two years. That was a weekly group session with six other guys and a couple of psychologists. Just being able to take a step back, to be curious – that's one of the big components of that. How am I feeling like that? All of it is to do with relationships. Instead of getting black or white thinking. they call it, you go "I'm going to have to check this out with the other person." It's so easy to miscommunicate, to get things mixed up, and if we're not careful we can go off the wrong way. So that was a big turning point.

Another massive turning point was when my grandson was born last year, and that was amazing – just wonderful. And my own children and my family as a whole, they've been such a massive support – just to realise that they love me, they accept me, they understand me and just to hold on to that gratefulness, is a massive turning point. And just to realise that this is a part of my life, it's not my whole life and there's life after being in hospital.

Is there anything else you want to add?

Aye, just to say how grateful I am for the help that I've had, from everybody. From fellow patients, from staff, advocacy, Patients Council. It's reassuring that there are people there who are interested. Who care. And just that encouragement, what a difference that makes – because there are times that it's been a very lonely experience.

It's not something I would have chosen – definitely not – but I have learned a lot from it, I have made a lot of good friends and I've had a lot of help, and hopefully I've helped people too. The way I like to look at it is, the second part of my life will be a lot better. The first part of my life, as I say, it was really good. A lot of things started going not so well but the second part, I'm looking forward to it. Just to be with my family and my friends and hopefully through time, I will be able to help other people – because it is a lonely place to be and as I say, it's just realising that there is hope.

> *There's always hope. Never give up, that's the most important. Never give up, there's always hope. There's always hope.*

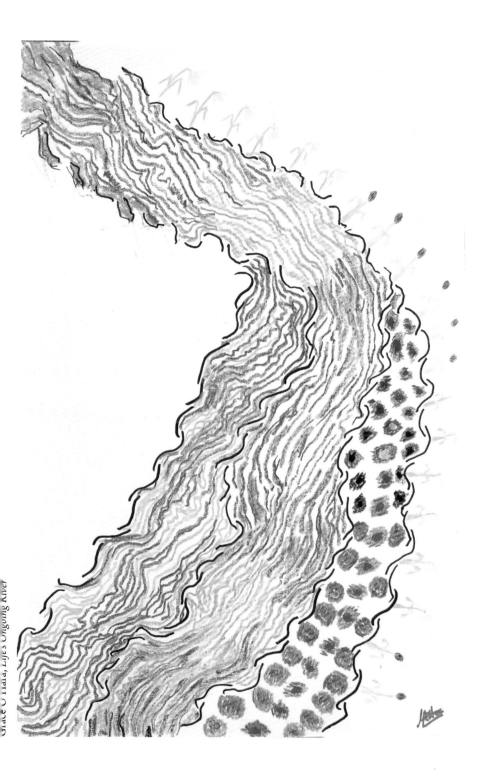

DOUGIE SOUTAR

Life is Never Boring

Stuck in this Hostel, all day long
God it's so boring, that's why I've got this song
Been here so long now, I've stuck to the floor
God it's so boring, can't take it no more.

Stuck at Sprout Market, turfing all day
God it's so boring, don't know why I stay
I've been here so long now, I'm stuck in the soil
God it's so boring, this kettle won't boil.

Stuck in the Royal Ed., singing this song
A recurring illness, recovery is long
I've been here nine times now, with each passing phase
God it's so boring, this drug-induced haze.

Working for Sam H, for hours every day
This hot and cold office, with people to pay
It's only some numbers, these millions of pounds
I just pay the wages, the staff do the rounds.

Stuck at the Stafford Centre, playing this song
The pool table's boring, so I've got this song
Playing in the music group, with Derek and Tom
It's no longer boring, we play all these songs.

Brahma Kumaris, is where I am now
I've learned meditation, my mind is quite sound
Now God isn't boring, we call Him our friend
It's been a long journey, with Peace in the end.

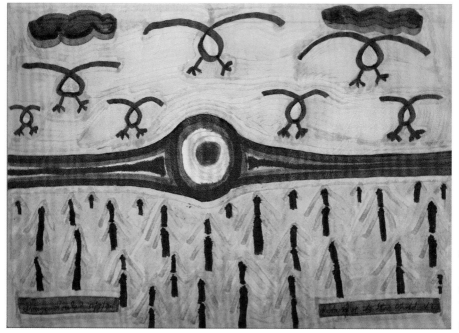

(a) As a student when I came to Edinburgh, my life's ambition was to see the sunrise. A symbol of rebirth.

(b) I traced back the origin of the bird design, to a TV program showing storks nesting on roofs in either Netherlands or Germany. Basic shape of the birds is a symbol of freedom.

(c) The forest trees are Douglas firs, and also a story from Shakespeare's Macbeth.

(d) The drawing here is a re-working of an original painting by myself on my first of many visits to REH, around 1977.

ACKNOWLEDGEMENTS

Thanks are due to a huge number of people who made this project possible:

To the editors of volumes one and two, Lesley Smith and Ronnie Jack.

To Isla Jack, for the foreword written in memory of Ronnie Jack.

To creative partners and workshop leaders Margaret Drysdale, Peter E. Ross (Chiaroscuro), Anne Elliot (Artlink), and Lilli Fullerton & Pam van de Brug (CAPS).

To members of the partners' group, Cat Young and Linda Irvine (NHS Lothian), and Jane Crawford (CAPS).

To our funders, the NHS Lothian Mental Health Strategy – A Sense of Belonging

To the staff of the Royal Edinburgh Hospital who supported the project, including the rehabilitation ward charge nurses, Mo Sofio and the Community Rehabilitation Team, and Claire Martin (OT).

To the Patients Council subcommittee members who provided support and guidance: Alison Robertson, Patricia Whalley, Stephen Muirhead, and Martin McAlpine.

To the Volunteer Hub for use of the lovely Library space at the hospital, and for putting us in touch with a volunteer transcriber.

To Katie Innes, for transcribing two interviews with skill and speed.

To the Scottish Mental Health Arts and Film Festival, for a grant to launch the book and create an exhibition.

To Pam van de Brug and CAPS, for support with the exhibition and launch venue.

To Patients Council staff Simon Porter and Maggie McIvor for invaluable day to day support and guidance.

To Albie Clark (Artlink) for designing the book with skill and patience.

And most importantly, to the contributors, without whose generosity there would be no book at all.